YOUR SKIN AND THE SUN

YOUR SKIN AND THE SUN

HOW TO PROTECT YOUR SKIN IN OUR CHANGING ENVIRONMENT — A GUIDE FOR THE WHOLE FAMILY

DR ANTHONY EMMETT

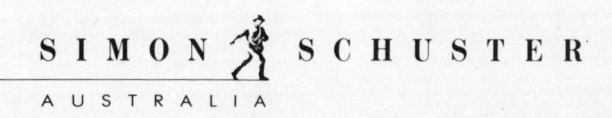

SIMON SCHUSTER
AUSTRALIA

YOUR SKIN AND THE SUN

First published in Australasia in 1990 by
Simon & Schuster Australia
7 Grosvenor Place, Brookvale NSW 2100

A Paramount Communications Company
Sydney New York London Toronto Tokyo Singapore

© 1990 Dr Anthony J. J. Emmett

All rights reserved. No part of this publication may
be reproduced, stored in a retrieval system, or
transmitted, in any form or by any means,
electronic, mechanical, photocopying, recording or
otherwise, without the prior permission of the
publisher in writing.

National Library of Australia
Cataloguing in Publication data
Emmett, Anthony J. J.
    Your skin and the sun : a passport to skin care
    in the nineties.

    Includes index.
    ISBN 0 7318 0177 6.

    1. Skin. 2. Solar radiation — Physiological
    effect. 3. Ultraviolet radiation — Physiological
    effect. 4. Suntan. I. Title.

646.726

Designed by Chris Hatcher/Graphix
Illustrated by Roger Roberts
Typeset in Australia by Post Typesetters
Printed in Australia by Australian Print Group

Contents

Introduction 7
Chapter 1. Our Changing Environment 9
Chapter 2. Learning About Your Skin 15
Chapter 3. Methods of Sun Protection 23
Chapter 4. Sunburn and its Treatment 35
Chapter 5. The Value of Sunglasses 41
Chapter 6. The Sun on Your Lips 45
Chapter 7. Moles, Sun Spots and Skin Cancers 51
Chapter 8. Caring for Your Skin 63
Chapter 9. Other Effects of Strong Sunshine 73
Chapter 10. Living Without the Sun 77
Appendix The Structure of Light 81
Index 85

Introduction

We are becoming more aware these days of the need to stay out of the sun. In recent years, the number of people with skin cancer and other skin complaints has been increasing to an alarmingly high level. This book warns us of the dangers of overexposure to sunlight. We need to become aware of the effects of sunlight on our skin, both in the short and long term. This book explains how to take appropriate steps to change our lifestyles.

The effects of the sun are cumulative so it is very important that children right from birth are protected and encouraged to develop lifelong habits avoiding overexposure to the sun.

Old habits are hard to change, but as the climate seems to be changing due to the Greenhouse Effect and the protective ozone layer around the Earth has been damaged, allowing increased levels of harmful radiation to reach Earth, we have to seriously reconsider our lifestyles.

With the greater incidence of skin cancer, we are now questioning the importance of a tan. For the past sixty years fashion has dictated a tan. Now the results of this can be seen everywhere — prematurely aged, wrinkled complexions, and young people, not just the aged, with life-threatening skin cancers.

Different skin types need different levels of protection so this book describes the characteristics of various skin types and recommends appropriate precautions we can take. With greater mobility and leisure time than that enjoyed by previous generations, we now have more opportunities to expose ourselves to the sun. It is vital that we be aware of the limitations of our own skin type.

As skin damage to a greater or lesser extent is common, this book also provides advice on skin care and surgical remedies. It shows us how to live a healthy life aware of the danger of the sun.

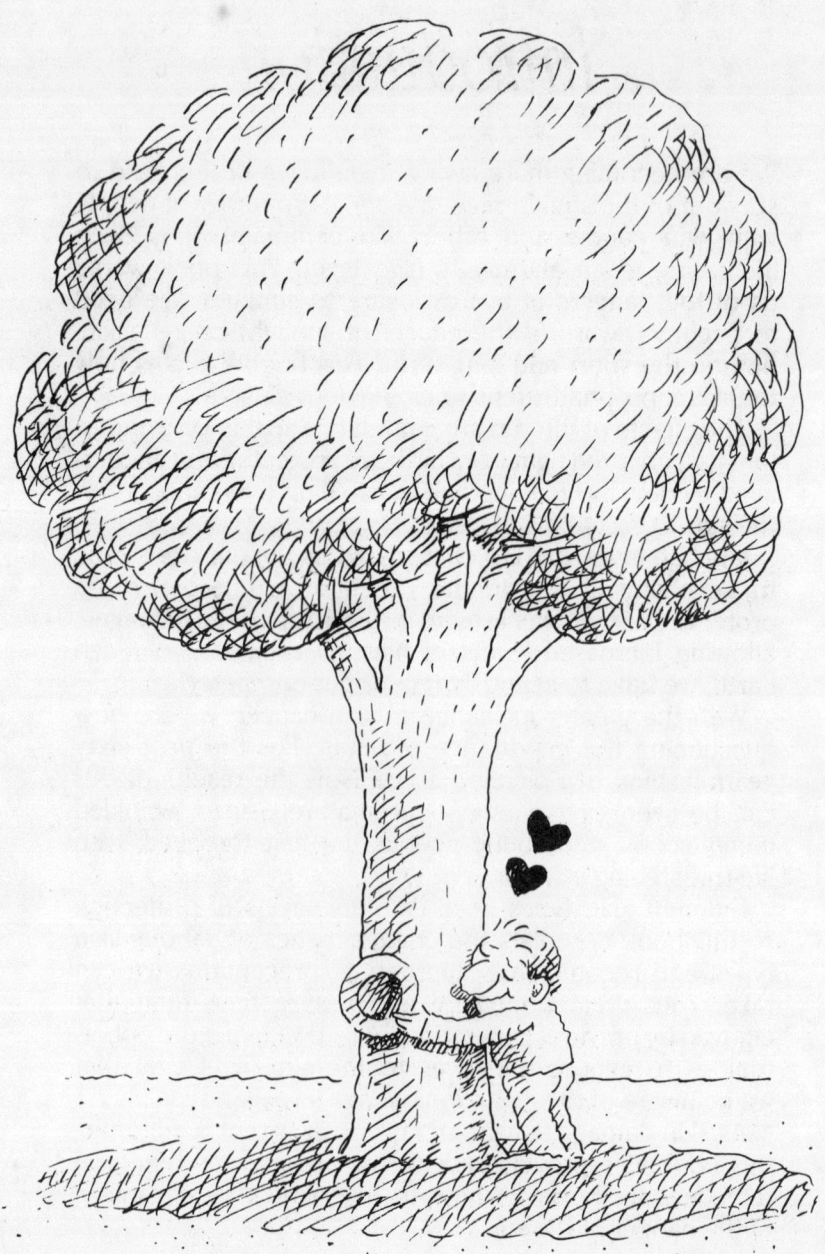

CHAPTER *1*

Our Changing Environment

We live in a time when many things are perceived to be changing. These changes have come upon us gradually and involve many aspects of our lives. We have much greater freedom in terms of the ability to travel easily with petrol or diesel engines and jet engines in aeroplanes. At the same time we are more crowded as there have never been so many people living on Earth.

For centuries we have been cutting down our forests to make ships, houses, furniture, firewood and so on, and our rate of replanting has always been inadequate. Even in ancient Egypt at the time of the Pharaohs, the Egyptians became short of timber from felling their forests and had to import it from nearby countries. Since then, this sorry situation has been repeated many times. The timber to construct the Spanish Armada and the oak that was used to build the victorious British warships at Trafalgar came from oak forests which no longer exist. Population pressure combined with mounting demand on scarce natural resources is bringing profound changes to our planet.

How does it all affect us? The common perception of a luxurious life includes a sun deck, water sports, a yacht and the time to enjoy them. Sunshine has become the epitome of warm happiness. At the same time, fair-skinned people are suffering skin cancers in ever-increasing numbers and in some parts of the world these have reached epidemic proportions. What we do not know is whether this is simply due to our lifestyle and the affluence of the present generation that enables us to spend more time in the sun when our skins are frequently unsuited to it, or whether there is a basic change in the atmosphere that is allowing more of the damaging rays of sunlight through to our skins.

THE OZONE LAYER

We know that the ozone layer in the upper atmosphere filters out the higher energy ultraviolet radiation. Ultraviolet radiation is invisible but it still comes along with the visible light from the sun. It will penetrate cloud cover and still affects the skin even though the day may not be hot or bright.

Ultraviolet-C (UV-C) is the highest energy ultraviolet. (See Appendix — Structure of Light.) Ultraviolet-C normally does not reach the surface of the Earth as it is all filtered out.

Ultraviolet-B (UV-B) is the ultraviolet which is causing most skin cancers at the present time.

Ultraviolet-A (UV-A) is a lower energy ultraviolet which was once thought to be harmless but is now recognised as causing premature ageing of the skin and a predisposition to the effects of Ultraviolet-B in causing skin cancers.

We know that there have been changes in the ozone layer and satellite photographs and gas samples from high-flying aeroplanes have shown that there are seasonal holes which have been forming in the last few years in the Southern Pacific in relation to the Antarctic.

What we do not know is whether or not these cyclical changes have been going on for a long time or whether they represent a permanent change which is the result of the use of chloro-fluoro-carbon (CFC) gases as propellants, refrigerants, and in the manufacture of plastics.

We have to assume, however, that changes are taking place and we are going to need to take more care with regard to protecting our skins from ultraviolet radiation in the future.

THE GREENHOUSE EFFECT

The so-called Greenhouse Effect is due to rising carbon dioxide levels which are associated with more consumption of oxygen and less production of it. Large amounts of forest have been destroyed over many centuries and this is happening more and more in various parts of the world, particularly in the Amazon Basin. Destruction of forests results in a reduced production of oxygen by the process of photosynthesis in which trees take in carbon dioxide using the energy of sunlight and create vegetable matter with oxygen as a by-product.

All green things use photosynthesis and this is the basic energy cycle on which we all depend for the production of fruits, vegetables, grain and other things we live on. The fish in the ocean feed on plankton that photosynthesise in the sea. The stored energy of oil and coal came from photosynthesis of plants many, many thousands of years ago.

The huge number of humans and their domestic animals existing on Earth are breathing in oxygen and breathing out carbon dioxide. At the same time, carbon dioxide is being produced from decomposing material and by-products of animal life generally. The enormous number of motorcars and trucks around the world are constantly consuming large quantities of oxygen as they burn petrol and diesel fuel in their engines.

The increasing carbon dioxide in the atmosphere is said to result in a warming of the planet and certainly we are seeing warmer summers in various parts of the world including Britain and Europe. Winters, too, are unseasonably warm.

Climatic changes combined with a more leisurely lifestyle

leave us more vulnerable to excessive exposure to the harmful rays of the sun.

THE SOCIAL TAN

It is important that we reassess our attitudes towards the so-called healthy life. It is now some sixty years since the tan became fashionable in the 1920s and 1930s. Before then, the tan was common only in manual workers and sailors and never in ladies or gentlemen. Two things contributed to that change of attitude. The first was that fashionable people like Coco Chanel in Paris began to exhibit a tan and many northern Europeans began to believe that the tan was a sign of health. Ultraviolet light had been used successfully to treat tuberculosis of the skin; it was also most effective for killing bacteria, so sunlight was considered healthy and a tan a natural extension of this idea. Whole sections of the population over the next thirty years set about making themselves brown in more and more areas of the body. Finally, today we see people with overall tans, with areas of the body such as the bottom and breasts which were once always white now being exposed to the sun, and gradually developing looser, wrinkled skin.

APPEARANCE

Because fair-skinned people in hot climates do not have pink cheeks they seek a tan to give colour to their skin. In the colder regions from which the white races came, the colder winter results in pink cheeks. Cold weather causes small blood vessels in the cheeks' skin to open more and so warm the skin, and this produces a blush. In the absence of the cold, this does not happen. This is also the reason why the tan which comes from snow-skiing has a different colour from the tan which comes from lying on the beach. The snow-ski tan has the pink cheek beneath it which gives it a more rosy brown colour.

YOUNG PEOPLE

It is a myth that it is more healthy and sexually attractive to have a brown skin rather than a white one. There is a great desire for young people to conform, to have a tan to fit in with their crowd, and they ignore the fact that their skin may not be able to tan at all. They will burn and freckle and spoil their complexion in a vain attempt to be brown.

Young skin is more susceptible for reasons that we don't fully understand, but presumably because the cells of the skin in a young person are multiplying more rapidly as they grow. We know that when cells are multiplying rapidly, they are more sensitive to X-rays (another form of invisible radiation) and to ultraviolet.

People who have spent their youth in the sun in countries like Australia, New Zealand, Africa and the southern United States, age more quickly in their thirties and forties than people who have spent their youth in a cold, non-sunny climate.

People who have spent their youth in a sunny climate and then move to a non-sunny climate have a higher incidence of melanoma than those people who have always been in that non-sunny climate.

BABIES

There is a feeling in Europe that it is good to put the baby out in the sun and fresh air. That may be acceptable practice when there is a dense atmosphere overlying which is filtering out much of the ultraviolet radiation from the sun and the sun's rays are coming obliquely through the Earth's atmosphere so that it is a very weakened sunlight that is reaching the baby.

In more sunny climates, the rays of the sun are much stronger and are definitely quite damaging to children's skin. Damage in the first ten years of life is much more significant than later. Remember that you do not want your child to end up with a wrinkled, prune-like skin by the age of thirty, nor to be prone to the development of future skin cancers. A given time of sun exposure is much more damaging to the child's skin than an equivalent exposure to the adult skin.

IS THE TAN SO HEALTHY THEN?

We know that many people form skin cancers of various types (discussed later in this book) and these may not only be crippling but also killing. We know that a tan causes premature ageing of the skin with wrinkling and loss of attractiveness.

We now know that, not only does ultraviolet radiation cause abnormal or malignant cells to develop in the skin, but it also retards the immune response that would normally be able to dispose of those cells. This crippling of the immune response is not limited to the skin but is also seen in the white blood cells in the body which become less able to withstand disease as a result of ultraviolet radiation. The "healthy" tan is not so healthy after all.

We do know that a certain amount of ultraviolet radiation is necessary for the production of Vitamin D to withstand the disease rickets which causes softening of the bones. The amount needed is really quite small though and in tropical countries there is enough reflected ultraviolet rays available to provide this without direct sunlight. Vitamin D can also be taken as a dietary supplement.

Though sunshine and good weather are to be appreciated, we have to dispel the myths that exposure to sunshine is essential to long-term good health. At last advertising and fashion promotions feature people with clear, pale skins. Sportsmen and women, our popular heroes, are setting an example by wearing hats and other protective clothing while playing sport. Our skin needs to be protected and the sun respected.

CHAPTER *2*

Learning About Your Skin

An understanding of skin types will help us to appreciate the problems of overexposure to the sun and to place a high value on our skin and its importance for good health. All around the world, people have developed many different skin types to suit different climatic zones. In Africa and the countries on either side of the equator, the black skin of the Negro is not only heavily pigmented but also reasonably thick and greasy. The pigment melanin is a natural sunscreen and it lies initially in the epidermis or cellular layer of the skin where it is formed and then passes upwards to lie in the horny outer layer of the skin where it can protect the active cellular epidermis from ultraviolet radiation. Even a Negro skin will become darker when exposed to sunlight and will become lighter if it is protected from the sun.

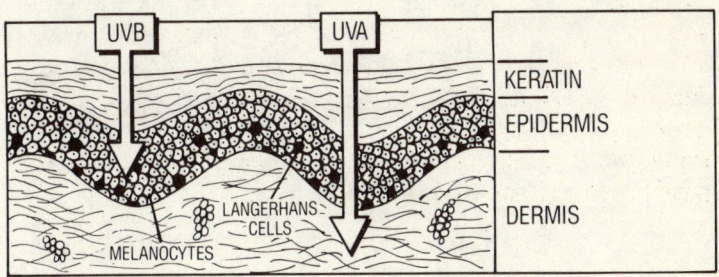

Layers of the skin

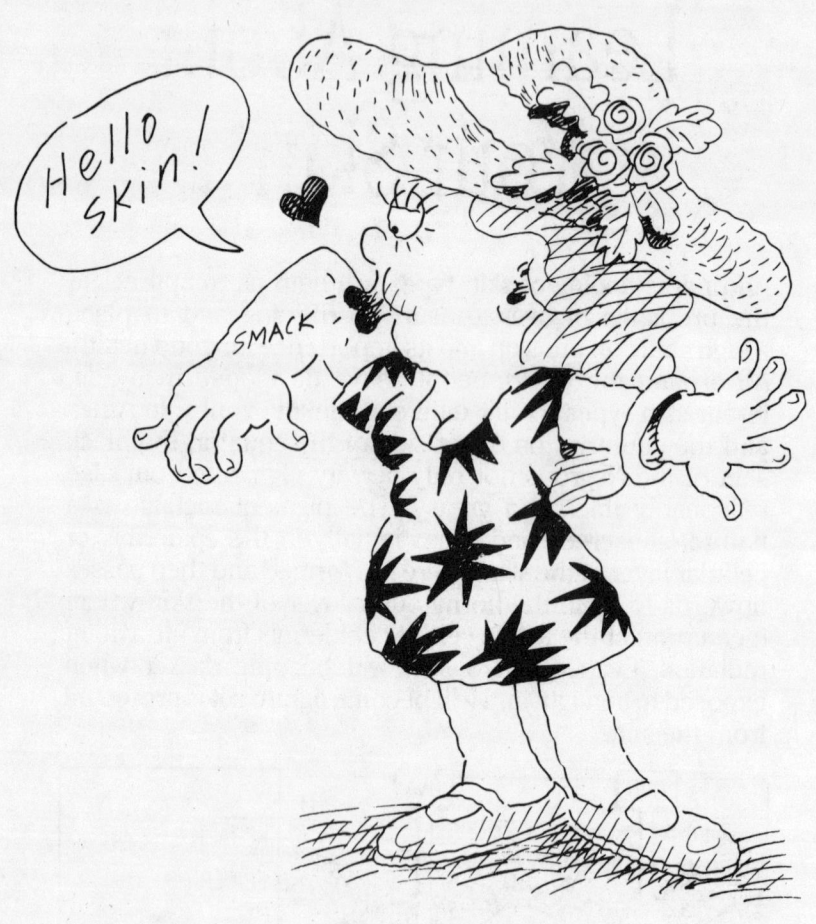

Fine, fair, dry skin has developed in Northern Europe in areas where sunshine is scarce and there is a necessity to absorb as much ultraviolet radiation as possible to form Vitamin D and prevent the disease rickets. These skins stay as fair as possible and actively shed pigment so that people who have this Type I fair skin find it impossible to hold a tan and are most subject to damage from ultraviolet radiation.

SKIN TYPES

For convenience in discussion, skin types are classed I to VI.

Type I: Sensitive skin which always burns easily and will not tan.

Type II: Sensitive skin which burns but will tan minimally.

Type III: Normal skin which burns moderately and tans slowly.

Type IV: Normal skin which burns minimally and tans well.

Type V: Skin that is resistant to sunshine, rarely burns and tans with vigour.

Type VI: Skin that is resistant to sunshine, never burns and is deeply pigmented.

Type I skin may take six to nine minutes to produce early sunburn on unprotected skin.

Type II skin is a little less sensitive than Type I but will tan a little more and not burn quite as quickly.
  The complexion of a person having Type I or II is usually fair. There may be freckles present and the hair colour may be blond, light brown or red.

A person with skin Type III will burn moderately and tan slowly. It takes longer for a Type III skin to become sunburnt and the unprotected skin may require about twelve minutes exposure to produce early sunburn. This will vary, of course, with different latitudes and times of the year. Type III skins are starting to become olive, a little greasier and more comfortable with the sun.

The more olive-skinned type of person is Type IV. The skin is often a little thicker and a little greasier. It is a skin that generally handles the sun quite well and people with this type of skin are often surprised when, after years of exposure, they start to show inevitable signs of damage. Type IV may be the Mediterranean type of skin often seen in southern Italians and Greeks as well as Turks and Spaniards.

Type V skins are darker and oilier and this type of skin can be found in Arabic, Oriental and Mediterranean peoples such as Spaniards, Turks, Greeks and southern Italians. As with Type IV, this type of skin will remain lighter when kept out of the sun and can become quite dark when exposed progressively over a period of time.

Type VI skin is darkest in colour and typically involves the Aboriginal or the Negro but may also involve other groups such as people from the Sudan, Ethiopia, Melanesia and Polynesia. There is a variation within these groups and some of them may be Type V or Type VI depending on tribal patterns.

CELTS' SKIN

Those of Celtic origin are most sensitive to the sun. The Celtic gene seems to carry with it a particular predisposition to skin cancer and even when a Celt has interbred with a heavily-pigmented person, it appears the tendency to skin cancer remains. The Celts were widely spread through Europe and are to be found in northern Germany, France, England, Scotland and especially Ireland. Ireland has the highest proportion of Celts and, per head of population, skin cancers are more common in Ireland than they are in England which is at a similar latitude but with a different racial grouping.

INDIVIDUAL SKIN PERFORMANCE

We live in a world where people are expected to have a tan as part of looking well and if someone is pale, they are likely to be asked "Are you sick?" This is unfortunate because it encourages people who cannot tan to try to do so with the inevitable consequence of later skin damage. For each individual it is necessary to be aware of one's own skin performance.

Parents need to observe their children and realise which of them are sun-sensitive and which are sun-resistant. It often happens that even in the same family one or two children will be very fair-skinned and sun-sensitive and one or two will be quite well-pigmented and better able to handle the sun.

At times you will find a fair-skinned, sun-sensitive woman married to an olive-skinned, easily-pigmenting man with both of them expecting to do the same recreational activity in the sun. The fair-skinned person will need, as much as is possible, to have a different lifestyle from the darker-skinned person, the fair-skinned person needing to avoid the sun. Where avoidance of the sun is not possible, it will be necessary to apply sunfilters more painstakingly, to see that the filter is applied at least half an hour before sun exposure begins, to reapply the filter as often as necessary to maintain a good thickness of film, to wear protective clothing, and to avoid the middle part of the day when the sun's rays are most intense. For fair-skinned people, this comes as a great imposition and it is easy to see why many do not take such precautions either through embarrassment of a perceived weakness, or laziness or just preferring to ignore it.

JOBS AND OCCUPATIONS

The very fair-skinned person, notably a Type I or II, needs to consider an indoor job or a job in a shaded area in preference to a job which involves working in the direct rays of the sun.

At times this can be difficult, such as when a sun-sensitive individual is thinking of purchasing a farm. This person would need to be counselled as to what will be involved in the long term as well as considering ways of avoiding skin problems, such as by ploughing the fields by night with a tractor fitted with floodlights, or using an air-conditioned cab with sunfilter glass in the daytime.

In guiding children towards an occupation, perhaps parents and teachers need to bear in mind the skin type of the child as well as their intellectual and manual abilities.

GUIDELINES FOR SKIN CARE

The determining factor in how long to remain in the sun is decided by skin type, time of day, latitude and climatic conditions. Thus, in the area adjoining the equator where the sun's rays travel most directly through the atmosphere and are least filtered, it is at the middle of the day that the sun's intensity is greatest and there will be maximum ultraviolet radiation. In the early morning and late afternoon the sun's rays pass obliquely through the Earth's atmosphere providing a greater filtering effect and reducing the intensity. As one climbs to higher altitudes, there is less atmospheric filtering of the rays and they become stronger. This is particularly so where there is a strong reflection of sunlight from snow, sand or water. While a heavy cloud cover will reduce the ultraviolet penetration, it does not stop it. Similarly, a layer of smog in heavily industrialised countries will also act as a sunfilter, limiting ultraviolet penetration, but still not stopping it.

Despite the fact that time of day, geographic location and atmospheric conditions are important, the most important factor of all is skin type. Those population groups from Northern Europe, Scotland and Ireland who have migrated to sunnier regions have paid the price for relishing the sunny climate by forming many skin cancers and other sun-induced skin conditions. Nevertheless, those who have stayed behind also form many skin cancers and one sees in clinics in Scotland and Ireland exactly the same types of skin cancer, although not in as high numbers or with the florid development that has been reached in the new world.

IS THERE A SAFE TAN?

It is vital to realise that there is no such thing as a safe way to tan. Solariums have been popular — they enable people to tan under lamps producing Ultraviolet-A (UV-A). However, it is now recognised that UV-A damages the immune system, ages the skin and worsens the effect of UV-B which produces skin cancers.

Exposing the skin to sun for only a few minutes daily over many weeks will produce a tan without burning. However, skin damage will still occur.

THE FUTURE

Those fair-skinned people who have migrated to sunnier regions and have made a new permanent home often wonder if their own sun exposure is going to improve the performance of that of their children in terms of skin response to the sun.

It is true that racial groups have modified their skin type in adapting to their region of the world. This, however, has taken many thousands of years. It is probably true to say that in the foreseeable future those with sun-sensitive fair skins will have children who also have this problem. Interbreeding with a more heavily pigmented partner is the most rapid way to produce more suitable skin types for sun exposure, but the children will have a mixture of darker and lighter skin type and the result will not be uniform. Some will have well-pigmented skins but their brothers and sisters may be fair.

Remember that the Moors from Africa resided in Spain for some four hundred years and their legacy was the darker skin of the Spaniard. Some of the Spaniards wrecked on the Irish coast after the Armada was scattered interbred with the Irish producing the darker-skinned Irish with blue eyes. These darker-skinned Irish still have the Celtic gene and a strong tendency to skin cancers, despite the pigmentation.

In the future, then, fair-skinned people will still need to protect themselves from excessive sun exposure and modify their lives according to their geographic location, skin type, occupation and pleasurable pursuits.

We may hope that genetic engineering will some day help to train melanocytes (pigment cells) to better protect fair and sensitive skins, and also help to modify the skin's immune protection system to resist the onslaught of ultraviolet radiation.

CHAPTER 3

Methods of Sun Protection

For those of us who have fair skins, learning how to avoid damage from the rays of the sun is vital. If you and your family live in a sunny climate, there are many small things you can do that will help. While it is true that the most important thing is the regular use of sunfilters, there are still many other things you can do as well.

CLOTHING AND ACCESSORIES

If you are going to be out in the sun, try to wear clothing that will protect your body and limbs from the penetration of ultraviolet radiation. The cloth must be sufficiently dense and you should avoid the porous, open weave cloth that allows the sun to shine through. Alternatively, if you want some sun to come through, that porous cloth can be quite a good medium sunfilter.

Long sleeves will protect the forearm and cotton gloves can be worn to protect the back of the hand. Long trousers will protect your knees and thighs as well as calves but the back of the foot also needs protection and a suitable casual shoe with or without socks will protect the feet.

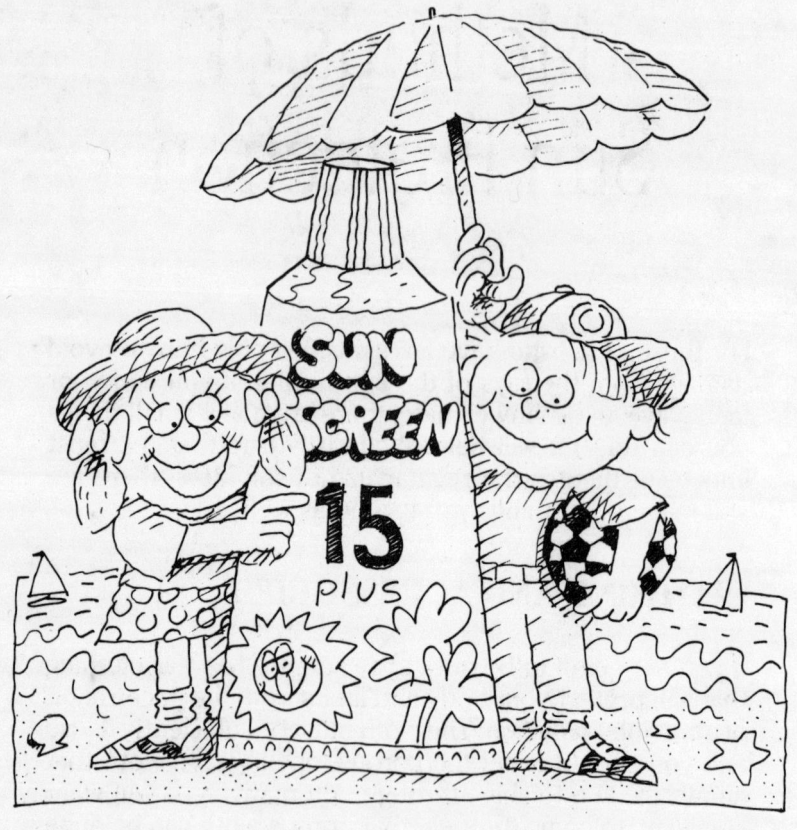

Turn your collar up to protect the back of the neck and button up the shirt to protect the front of your chest.

If you or your children are going swimming at the beach or an outdoor pool, a shirt can be worn in the water to protect from sunlight and it has now been shown that getting the shirt wet does not increase the penetration of ultraviolet as long as the weave is sufficiently close. After you have been swimming you may be sitting under a beach umbrella and you should then put on protective clothing to prevent ultraviolet rays that reflect up off the sand from affecting you. Likewise, when boating, you should be careful to avoid burning from rays reflected from the water.

GLOVES

The back of the hand is a common site of solar keratoses and skin cancers which come from many years of exposure to sunshine. Wearing cotton gloves is a very effective method of protection. The backs of the hands are especially vulnerable when gardening, playing sport and driving a car.

HATS

Hats have many uses in different climates at different times. In very cold climates, thicker hats are worn to keep the head warm, while in hot climates broader-brimmed, porous hats are worn to deflect the sun and to allow the head to remain cool. Hats are protection too.

Hats are in fashion for outdoor wear and these can be cooling but it is desirable that the brim should be sufficiently broad so that the ears are protected from the sun. We frequently forget to put sunfilter on the ears and on the skin behind the ear.

Most hats are not sufficiently broad-brimmed to protect the lips or the neck. The small towelling hat that many wear does not really protect the face from the sunshine.

Broader brims on the front and the back of the hat will tend to protect the neck more but a scarf or a sunfilter is usually necessary for additional neck protection.

THE PARASOL

The parasol or umbrella has been, in times past, an object of beauty and fashionable interest. The parasol still is a most effective way to keep cool and avoid the direct rays of the sun. Many types are available — from the Chinese version made of bamboo with waxed paper and beautiful decorations to the black umbrella of Europe or the beautifully patterned, light, nylon umbrellas. Even though one is wearing a hat, one can get much more shade with a parasol or umbrella and it could be time that these came back into favour as a fashion accessory that is beneficial for your skin.

SOAP AND WATER

If you are planning to spend a day in the sun, it is probably better that you wash in the evening rather than in the morning because in this way there is more oil left on the skin. It is also better to shave in the evening as hair and a thicker outer skin layer act as filtering agents. Shaving removes some outer layer skin and grease, as well as hair.

Sunfilters are best applied early in the morning well before going into the sun and starting to perspire.

SUNSCREENS

Not only do people vary from one to another in their sensitivity to the sun but different parts of the body will also be variably sensitive. Those parts of the body which are not usually exposed to sunlight will often burn more easily than other areas more often exposed. This variation is related to the melanin pigment in the skin and also the thickness of the outer layer of the skin. Skins habitually exposed to the sun tend to have thicker outer layers.

PHYSICAL SUNSCREENS

These are an opaque film which will reflect or scatter the ultraviolet radiation before it reaches the skin. The best example of a physical sunscreen is zinc cream which forms a dense barrier on the skin but there is a limit as to how much of the body can be covered with it as it blocks perspiration. Generally, its use is limited to specific areas such as the nose, or lips. Calamine also can be an opaque physical filter.

Make-up also acts as an opaque filter because of the titanium oxide in many types of make-up. In addition to the physical barrier offered by make-up, it may also contain a chemical sunscreen.

Any opaque substance on the skin may be a physical sunscreen. Thus, dirt is the simplest sunscreen of all and, at times, a layer of dirt, ash or mud plastered onto the skin can be the simplest way of gaining protection. Australian Aborigines are said to have used this technique during the very hot sunny times.

CHEMICAL SUNSCREENS

These may be either a water-soluble or an oil-soluble chemical which will absorb ultraviolet radiation and reduce its intensity. These agents may be clear and can be applied to the skin in a variety of vehicles (creams, oils, and so on). They may be applied in an alcohol-based lotion which dries quickly and leaves the skin non-greasy, or as an ointment or a cream, or in make-up.

Sunscreens on the market initially were mainly absorbers of Ultraviolet-B but the newer broad-spectrum sunscreens also contain compounds which will absorb Ultraviolet-A. Previously, Ultraviolet-A was considered to be relatively harmless. Today, however, we look to see that a sunscreen will absorb both the Ultraviolet-A and the Ultraviolet-B and these are called *broad-spectrum sunscreens*. Their activity is generally graded according to their "sun protection factor" (SPF). Sunscreens are tested and allocated an SPF value which is determined by the amount of time they are able to extend an individual's ability to stay in the sun without burning. For example, a person who would normally burn after twelve minutes in the sun, by using an SPF10 sunfilter may extend that period of time to one hundred and twenty minutes before they will burn. SPF numbers have varied from 1 to 15 and we are now seeing numbers greater than 15 on sunfilter products.

Persons with sensitive skins are well advised to use the highest number SPF available. SPF numbers are generally allocated after testing the individual sunfilters, frequently using fair-skinned volunteers to determine the effectiveness of the product.

We need to consider the chemicals which are used as sunscreens and the vehicle in which they are carried. This vehicle can be a lotion which is quick drying, an ointment, cream, milk or a base which will withstand water and is useful to apply before swimming. Depending on your skin you may select different types of application.

Unfortunately there are no common names or symbols for the chemical sunscreens used in the various lotions and creams that are for sale by different manufacturers. The only way to find out what is in each one is to read the fine print on the bottle or tube.

The following chemical sunscreens will mainly filter out Ultraviolet-B.

Para-aminobenzoic	(PABA)
Diethanolamine p-methoxycinnamate	(Parsol hydro)
Ethyl 4-BIS hydroxypropyl-P aminobenzoate	(Amerscreen)
Ethylhexyl p-methoxycinnamate	(Parsol MCX)
2-ethylhexyl salicylate	(Octyl salicylate)
Homomenthyl salicylate	(Homosalate)
Octyl dimethyl p-aminobenzoate	(Padimate-0)
2-phenylbenzimidazole-5-sulfonic acid	(Eusolex 232)

(For example, Sea & Ski, Blockout, etc.)

There are also chemical sunscreens which will absorb Ultraviolet-A.

4-tert-butyl-4-methoxy-
dibenzoylmethane   (Parsol 1789)
4-tert-propyl-4-methoxy-
dibenzoylmethane   (Eusolex 8020)
(These are always combined with others and are not preparations on their own.)

Broad spectrum absorbers absorb Ultraviolet-A and Ultraviolet-B.

Dioxybenzone   (Benzophenone-8)
Oxybenzophenone   (Benzophenone-3)
Sulfisobenzone   (Benzophenone-4)
Complex mixture   (Eusolex 8021)
(For example, Roche, Eversun, Face Saver, etc.)

New sunscreens are being developed all the time. The important thing is to pick a screen which is broad-spectrum, absorbing Ultraviolet-A as well as Ultraviolet-B.

Seek advice from the chemist or your doctor if in doubt about which sunscreen to use.

SUNSCREEN APPLICATION

The effectiveness of a sunscreen will depend on the thickness of the layer which has been applied. The film should be even and it is important that it be applied well before going into the sun as perspiration will interrupt the evenness of the application. Some sunfilters are more effective if time is allowed for them to bond into the keratin or outer layer of the skin and this will take at least fifteen to thirty minutes.

Where water-resistant sunfilters are applied, these should again be applied half an hour before going into the water. Sunfilters will also need to be reapplied during the day, possibly every two or three hours depending on the type of activities engaged in and the amount of perspiration. This is necessary to maintain an even film of sunfilter or sunscreen.

An alcohol-based lotion (the alcohol can usually be smelt) containing a sunfilter has the advantage of being applied quickly and easily and is non-sticky as well as being clear and leaving the skin looking normal. However, this can be drying to an already dry skin and may be better avoided. Ointments, on the other hand, take longer to apply but if you have a dry skin they may be more suitable. Creams have more moisture and milks may be a compromise for dry skin allowing rapid application, while the sunfilter in make-up can be useful also.

Make sure that the sunfilter filters out the Ultraviolet-A as well as the Ultraviolet-B. When studying the list of ingredients on sunfilters before buying, you may find that some ingredients absorb Ultraviolet-A and others Ultraviolet-B or there may be an absorber which will absorb both A and B. It is then a matter of trying the preparation to see if it suits your skin, how easily it spreads and how well it appears to adhere to the skin.

SKIN REACTION

Not everybody is able to tolerate all of the various chemicals in sunfilters when applied to their skins. There will be some sunfilters that will suit you better than others. You will need to experiment when trying a cream, an ointment, or some other preparation to apply these substances to your skin.

At times when you have applied a sunfilter, you may find that it irritates your skin and in some people a phototoxic or photosensitising reaction can occur in which the chemical in the filter actually worsens the reaction to the sun. This is uncommon but it can happen in some people and when that is the case those ingredients must be avoided and a different type of sunfilter used. For this reason it is often worth buying a small quantity of the filter you are trying out initially to find whether or not it suits your skin.

SUNTANNING PREPARATIONS

In the tanning process, the initial brown appears as a result of the ultraviolet darkening melanin which is already present in the skin but has not yet developed its colour. This may develop in twelve hours and last for three to four days. On the other hand, it takes three or four days for new melanin to be produced after the ultraviolet exposure and it is about four to six days before this starts to appear as a tan which will go on increasing for three weeks. Further exposures will add more tan. While the tan is some protection against sunburn, the ultraviolet rays will still damage sensitive skin.

It needs to be noted that sunscreens do not promote the formation of melanin. However, there are compounds on the market which will promote a colouring of the skin although this colour may *not* be a protection against ultraviolet radiation. Chemicals such as dihydroxyacetone and tyrosine can cause the appearance of a tan. These quick-tanning preparations may also contain sunfilters and this should be described on the label. They may promote tanning in those who have difficulty but, again, must contain a sunscreen for protection.

MAKE-UP

Make-up has the advantage that one can provide immediate colour to the skin and the particles of titanium oxide pigment in the make-up are themselves a physical sunscreen. The addition of a chemical sunscreen to the make-up gives added protection, particularly when it is an Ultraviolet-A and B absorber. (For example, Elizabeth Arden and Clinique cover make-up.) In addition the make-up is a film which helps protect the skin from drying and it can be used with a moisturising cream as part of its foundation. Skilled advice by a beauty consultant on which make-up to use and which best suits your skin and general colouring is worthwhile before buying.

OTHER WAYS OF PROTECTION

DAILY HABIT

Perhaps one of the best means of sun protection is to get into the daily habit of doing outdoor things when the sun is at its weakest, and to do indoor work or indoor recreation when the sun is most intense.

Hanging clothes out on the clothesline in the early morning and taking them off in the late evening is a sensible routine. You may feel that this is going to fade the clothes but perhaps it is better to fade the clothes instead of damaging your skin. Alternatively, you could hang clothes out in the evening and bring them in next morning.

An electric clothes dryer avoids the necessity of turning your unprotected face up to the sun for the fifteen minutes that it takes to hang clothes on the line. Those fifteen minutes add up and in one year they come to quite a few minutes, that is, ninety hours, all of which is recorded in your skin.

RECREATION

Sporting fixtures also can be arranged to be held in the very early morning or late evening. Football fields, tennis courts and the like, need to be floodlit for night use. Sporting events in the middle of the day should be avoided or at least held in covered areas. Many people fail to take precautions to prevent skin damage while playing sport.

TREES, THE ENVIRONMENT AND YOUR SKIN

Trees are important in the environment to cleanse the air, lock up carbon dioxide, release oxygen and provide moisture. Not only beautiful, they also create much needed shade and coolness in hot weather. Swimming pools can be shaded by trees, as can car parks, footpaths and houses. Shaded, forested areas provide excellent recreation opportunities such as bushwalking and orienteering. Green leaves absorb ultraviolet rays whereas beaches, water and footpaths reflect it. The importance of trees to our health and well-being has been virtually ignored in the past. Now that we have to change our lifestyles to protect our skin from damage, trees will become invaluable.

CHILDREN'S SKIN

Children who have spent their childhood in a non-sunny climate have a reduced chance of getting skin cancers, particularly melanoma, when they move to a sunny climate (as compared with those children who grew up in that sunny climate). Even when children who grew up in sunny climates move to non-sunny climates, they still have an increased risk of all skin cancers, melanoma particularly, as compared with the inhabitants of the non-sunny region who spent their childhood there. This is because the effects of sun exposure are cumulative and progressive, so children are affected to a greater degree than adults.

The important message here is that every bit of sun protection that can be given to children is vital. It is worthwhile for them to wear hats on all possible occasions as well as protective clothing. Sunfilters should be used always on their exposed skin.

BABIES' SKIN

The skin of babies and young persons is sun-sensitive and they should never be placed in direct sunlight. Reflected sunlight is quite adequate and babies should be in the shade if placed outdoors, care being taken to see that, as the sun changes position, they are so placed that they avoid direct rays of the sun.

It is now recognised that the skin of babies is more sensitive to ultraviolet radiation than that of adults. Because the ultraviolet effect on the skin is permanent, care must be taken to prevent damage to the child's skin by early sun exposure. The simplest cover is a canopy over the pram. Use a sun hat, light but protective clothing, and if there is a great deal of reflected ultraviolet, then use a sunscreen as well. Remember not to leave your baby in a hot car and remember also that Ultraviolet-A comes through the glass of the car. Ultraviolet-B comes through open windows. Much skin damage occurs in cars and window shades are an important means of prevention.

Children in the sun require parental supervision to decide when they have had enough and which sunfilters and clothing, hats, and so on are to be used. For a given sun exposure of, say, fifteen minutes, the skin of a child will be more damaged than the skin of an adult although this effect may not show for many years.

MOTORCARS

It is easy to forget about sun protection while in a car. However drivers are at risk of skin cancers, particularly on the right cheek and temple, from the sun's radiation through the car window. Lips and the backs of hands are particularly vulnerable so protective clothing, sunscreens and hats are also important while travelling in cars. Protect the back seat with window shades.

CONCLUSION

Once you are aware of the sun and how it can affect you and your family, taking precautions to avoid skin damage becomes common sense. The difficult part is realising the pervasive nature of the sun's rays. This realisation is essential before changes in lifestyle with increased sun exposure become regular and permanent.

CHAPTER 4

Sunburn and its Treatment

Sunburn is caused by exposure to ultraviolet radiation which is itself invisible. It comes with the visible radiation from the sun and so on a bright, sunny day one is conscious of the heat, the light and the fact that the sun is affecting the skin. On the other hand, on a cloudy day when it's cooler, ultraviolet is still reaching the skin and can still cause a burn. Reflected ultraviolet may also reach the skin when one is in the shade.

The time it takes any one individual to become sunburnt will depend on the skin type and how much it is protected either by sunfiltering agents or by the presence of a tan or even by grease and dirt. Thus if you are a well-washed person with fair, dry skin, typical of Type I, who has no protective tan or sunfilter lotion, you are prone to burn very quickly. You would be unaware of the fact that your skin is being burned because of the delay period with ultraviolet radiation and would feel only a sense of warmth but no pain or discomfort. Unless you are aware that the "burn time" for that latitude and time of the year is, for example, twelve minutes for a fair-skinned person, your skin will be burnt before you feel any discomfort.

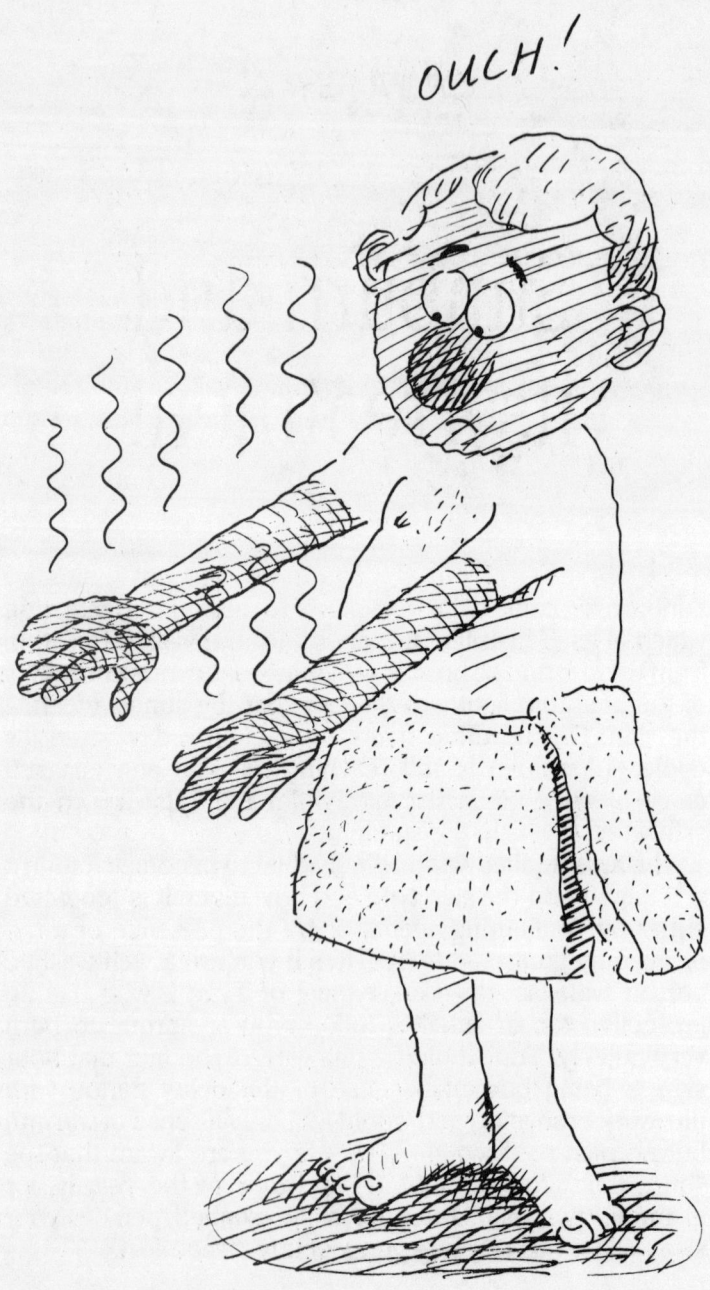

DEGREES OF SUNBURN

Sunburn can be classed as mild, moderate or severe.

Mild sunburn will begin some nine to twelve hours after the burning exposure and can be expected to fade in about twenty-four hours. A cold compress or a soothing lotion such as calamine may be applied or a cold bath can help. The sunburn is associated with the release into the tissues of a chemical "histamine" which contributes to the redness, swelling and pain and can also cause a headache. Antihistamine tablets can be helpful and an antihistamine cream can be used for direct application to the sunburnt area. Antihistamine tablets usually make one sleepy which can be welcome at such times, though newer antihistamines are available with less sedative effect if that is desired.

With *moderate sunburn,* the skin is a bright red. Treatment is similar to that for mild sunburn.

With *severe sunburn,* blisters will start to form one or two hours after exposure and will continue to increase for the first forty-eight hours. The swelling, redness and blisters may remain acute for the first five days and then will gradually settle over the next ten days or so. Treatment of severe sunburn is generally by cold compresses, cold baths and, at times, anaesthetic sprays. The addition of salt at the rate of one-half teaspoon per litre of water to the cold bath makes it more comfortable.

Medical advice is generally necessary at this stage and if there is any exposure of raw skin surface, then infection needs to be prevented. One agent which is in common usage is silver sulphadiazine, a white cream which is rubbed onto the surface once or twice a day, and washed off in a bath. This is generally used under medical supervision. Aspirin is useful for the reduction of both pain and inflammation, and antihistamines are also useful.

Treatment in hospital may be necessary and, with more extensive sunburns, replacement of fluid by intravenous transfusion can be prescribed as there is a considerable loss of fluid into the tissues of the body around the burnt area. This is usually required only in the first forty-eight hours. Healing is generally complete by two to three weeks except where the surface becomes infected and then there may be some scarring.

LATER EFFECTS OF SUNBURN

There are many later effects of sunburn quite apart from the pain and discomfort of the actual acute event.

There can be *pigmentary changes* in the skin which are semi-permanent. Sometimes these are lighter areas in which the melanocytes or tanning cells appear to have been permanently damaged and that particular piece of skin may have difficulty in browning. Sometimes this can be small, white, circular areas scattered through the burnt area, the so-called "white freckles"; at other times there may simply be an uneven pigmentation of the area.

Certainly, sunburn does leave its lasting effect in many people. It has been shown that in young people developing malignant melanoma, a history of intermittent episodes of sunburn can be traced over some years before the development of the melanoma. Sunburn, itself, appears to inflict considerable damage on the melanocytes which, normally, under a graduated sun exposure, would be responsible for producing the pigment in the skin to form a tan. Other cells in the skin are also injured by ultraviolet rays and these include the Langerhans cells which are part of the immune protection of the skin against the formation of skin malignancies. Areas of the body which have been subject to recurrent sunburn or strong sun exposure over the years are known to have a reduction in Langerhans cell numbers. This indicates reduced ability to withstand the formation of skin cancers.

PHOTOSENSITIVITY

This is a condition in which there is an over-response to sunlight resulting in a burn where it would otherwise not have been expected either to occur or to be that severe.

Agents which cause photosensitivity may be in some foodstuffs, some drugs, or some preparations that are applied to the skin.

Foodstuffs which contain psoralens or coumarins may cause photosensitivity in some people. These foods include parsnips, parsley, celery, anise, root vegetables, citrus fruits (including lime), rutaceae, bergamot, angelica, dill or fennel.

Some *drugs* may also cause photosensitivity. These include sulphonamides, halogenated salicylates and phenothiazines. Read all labels carefully.

A number of preparations applied to the skin surface can cause phototoxicity. Tars, for example, contain a variety of substances such as pyridine, anthracene and acridine which may cause this problem. Hexachlorophene, which is found in some soaps, detergents and shampoos, may also affect some people. The preparation 5-fluorouracil which is used in the treatment of some skin cancers of the superficial type is a marked photosensitiser and people receiving this treatment must avoid the sun.

Para-aminobenzoic acid (PABA) or its derivatives may be found in some sunscreen preparations and local anaesthetics and can cause photosensitisation in some people but this is uncommon. Some people also react to Cinnamic acid esters which are also used in sunscreens.

Dyes used in sunscreens, such as anthraquinone also have been known to photosensitise.

Many people today are using Retinoid derivatives (synthetic Vitamin A) to help retard or reverse some of the ageing effects of ultraviolet light on the skin and these substances are themselves photosensitisers while they are being used. It is important that all ultraviolet exposure must be avoided when using these derivatives.

AVOIDING SUNBURN

The best way to avoid sunburn is to be aware of your own skin's capacity to absorb ultraviolet radiation and, in particular, to know the measure of your "burn time". It is best to get into the habit of applying the sunfilter well before you go into the sun and to remember that a uniform thickness of sunfilter is important and that it can easily be rubbed or washed off during the day's activities. Reapplication every two or three hours is important as the thickness of the filtering agent determines its effectiveness.

Remember, also, that clothing such as long sleeves, long trousers and a good hat are a practical and economical protection. If you are going to have a day in the sun, it will be wise to shave in the evening rather than in the morning as this keeps a thicker outer (keratin) layer on your facial skin during the sunlight hours. A little extra grease and dirt may in themselves be beneficial.

Finally, be aware of the possibility that photosensitising (or phototoxic) reactions can occur especially if you are applying some new substance or eating some new food and then having a great amount of sun exposure. It is hard to predict this kind of reaction and the only way would be to try small test areas if in doubt and then to be cautious with sun exposure.

For the average person, thirty minutes of unprotected sun exposure will result in a painful redness while one full hour of exposure would produce a painful sunburn with redness and swelling. A two-hour exposure to the sun at its maximum intensity, that is, midday in midsummer, will produce sunburn with blistering taking seven to ten days to heal and leaving a spotty discolouration. Sunfilters need to be applied *fifteen to thirty minutes* before going out in the sun to achieve an even film on the skin. For those habitually in the sun, the filter is best applied in the early morning as part of routine toilet preparation. If washing or shaving in the morning, the sunfilter can be applied after that, before dressing.

Alternatively, simply apply the filter in the morning before dressing and bathe and/or shave in the evening.

CHAPTER 5

The Value of Sunglasses

The eye, of necessity, is exposed to the radiation of light and ultraviolet from the sun in all types of weather. Like the skin, the eye is affected by ultraviolet radiation but these effects are not immediately obvious. Important among these effects is the formation of a "cataract" which is an opacity which, over a number of years, develops in the lens of the eye. This has now been found to be related to ultraviolet exposure as well as to ageing.

In addition, a yellowish plaque (called pinguecula) can be formed because of a degeneration of the collagen fibres in the inner part of the white of the eye. With time, these may take on a fleshy look and may cover the central triangular white part of the eye, a condition called a pterygium. Sometimes these need surgery when they start to encroach on the clear area that is the cornea.

It can be difficult to protect the skin of the eyelids with sunfilters because they tend to run into the eye and irritate it particularly when one is hot and sweating or wet. There are make-up sticks for the eyelids containing sunfilters and these do not tend to run but they are rather awkward to use. The simplest way of protecting both eyes and the eyelids is with a pair of sunglasses that absorbs ultraviolet radiation.

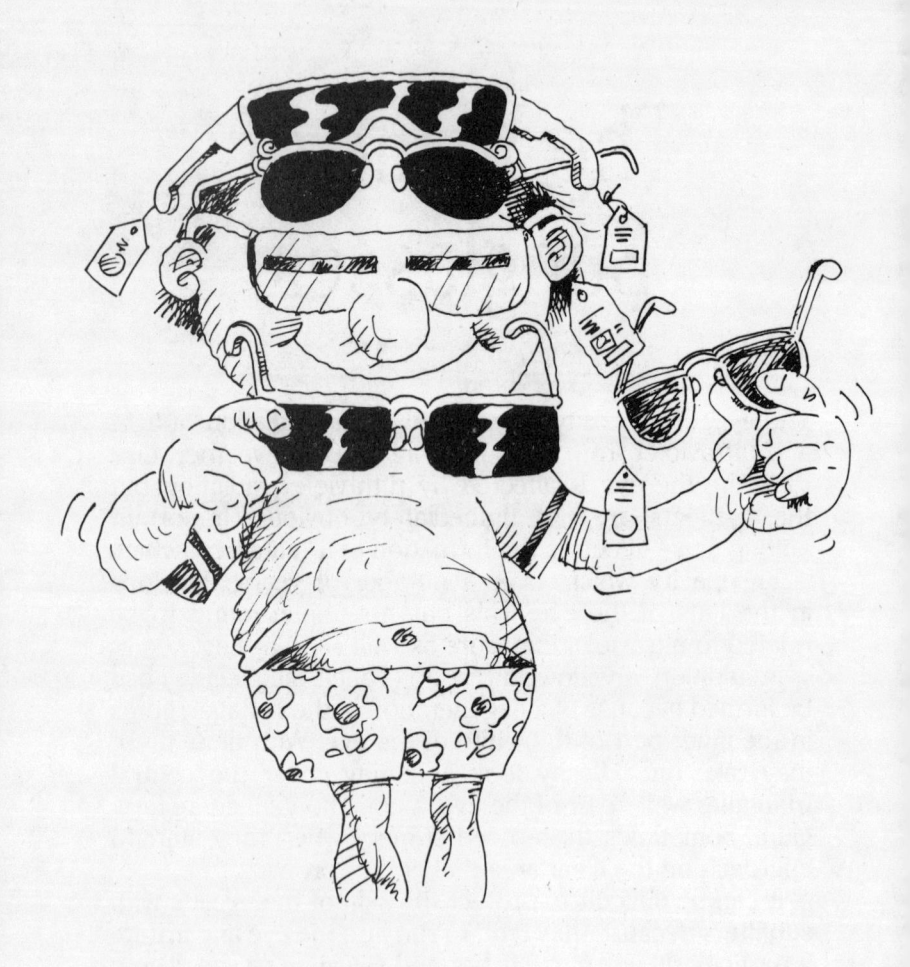

CHOOSING SUNGLASSES

The sunglasses that you buy should have a card attached to indicate which ultraviolet is absorbed. Sunglasses, when made of columbia resin (CR39), will filter to 360nm (nanometres or billionths of a metre) and, with additional ultraviolet absorbers, can filter to 400nm. As Ultraviolet-C is 200 to 280nm, Ultraviolet-B is 290 to 320nm and Ultraviolet-A is 320 to 400nm, it can be seen that filtering to 400nm will remove all of the A, B and C ultraviolet rays. (See Appendix — The Structure of Light.)

Good optical glass and polycarbonate lenses will both filter to 360nm. Metallic oxides used to tint glass can increase the absorbing and filtering effect further.

IMMEDIATE EFFECTS OF SUN ON THE EYE

In addition to the long-term effect of ultraviolet, one can also get a burn of the eye which is equivalent to sunburn resulting, after a few hours of exposure, in a feeling of irritation and grittiness with watering of the eye. Eyelid spasm can occur with the irritation. Soothing eyedrops and rest for the eye for forty-eight hours using protective eyepads and painkillers under medical supervision is the usual treatment.

It is important to be aware that the direct rays of the sun on the unprotected eye can cause these effects. One must remember never to look directly at the sun as this can cause permanent injury to the central sensitive part of the retina which is the seeing part of the eye. This damage can result in loss of parts of one's accurate vision.

EYELIDS

Eyelids, themselves, can form skin cancers particularly on the margin of the eyelid where it is impossible to put any kind of sunfilter. The only way to guard this area is with a sunfiltering sunglass. The sun may have other effects on the skin of the eyelid margin such as a chronic shortening of the skin as a long-term effect which can cause the eyelid margin to turn out. This can be corrected surgically if it occurs but is better avoided. Wrinkling and looseness of the eyelids due to loss of elasticity is another long-term sun effect.

WHEN TO WEAR SUNGLASSES

Sunlight effects accumulate in the eye as they do on the skin. When you are in high ultraviolet areas with intense light and reflection, always remember to protect your eyes with sunglasses. Remember, also, to protect the eyes of your young children as they, too, are sensitive to these radiations which will slowly and progressively affect them. Children are well advised to wear sunglasses whenever exposed to strong sunlight and this includes the trip to school when there is strong ultraviolet reflection from footpaths and roads. Hats are some protection for the eyes but do not interrupt the *reflected* ultraviolet radiation, so *appropriate* sunglasses are the answer for eyes that would be healthy.

CHAPTER 6

The Sun on Your Lips

The lip is exposed to sunlight more often than we realise and it is at great risk from reflected and direct ultraviolet radiation.

The sculptured fullness of the lips with the delicate curl out of the skin just above the red margin is one of the most treasured aspects of human beauty. There is, of course, an enormous variation in the shape of the lips and much has been written on the association between the shape of the lip and the personality of the individual. It is true that the muscle in the lip gives it much of its shape but the fine detail of contour comes from the skin structure at the lip edge. Where the skin turns out just before it becomes the red or vermilion border, there is a white roll of the skin edge which tends to be more marked in the upper lip than in the lower lip and in the upper lip this blends into the twin ridges of the central upper lip which are the columns of the philtrum. In many people this can be one of the most beautiful parts of the body but it is also one that is most readily damaged by the sun and its beauty destroyed. The collagen fibres of the dermis, that deeper part of the skin which gives it its strength, are responsible for the fine detail in this contour and it is these fibres which are damaged and aged by ultraviolet radiation from the sun.

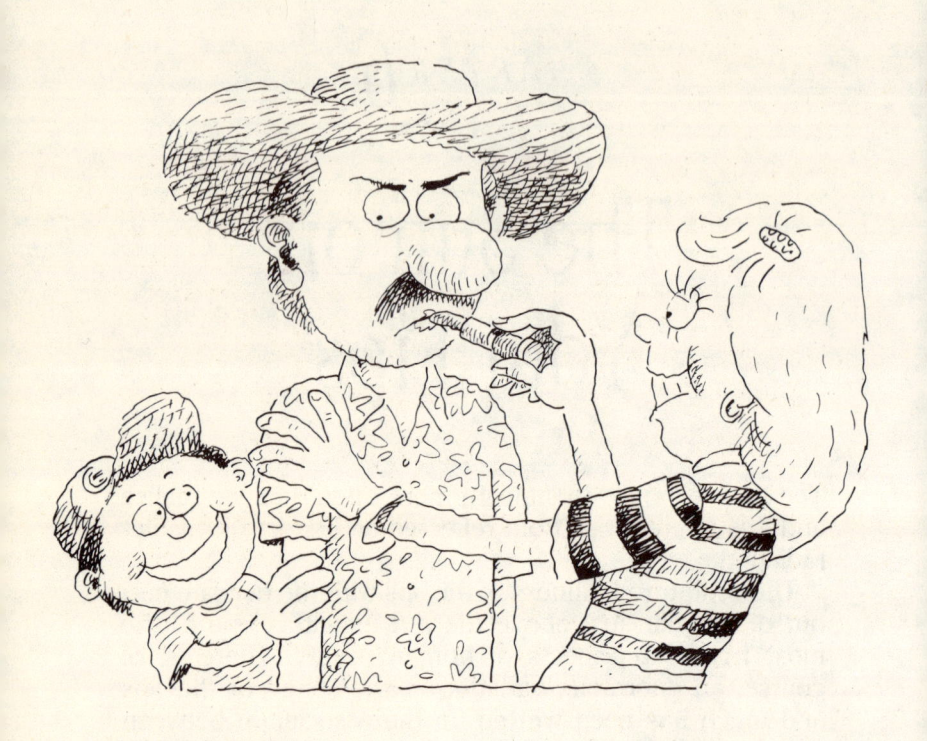

CHILDREN'S LIPS

When we look at the lips of a very young child, we see the expressive and generous fullness of the lip at its most beautiful. It is true that the shape of the lip changes as we grow and it often becomes a little less full and contoured, but, for those living a life out of the sun, the beauty of the lips can be retained into old age. On the other hand, those with steady sun exposure, especially in childhood, will be losing this beauty even by teenage and, by their mid-thirties, the attractive lip contours will be flattening and fading along with the elasticity of the skin. Remember the young lip, like the young skin, is *more affected* by a given time of sun exposure.

LIPS UNDER SUN EXPOSURE

Not only is the beauty of the lip lost, but there are also changes occurring in the red margin of the lip and skin, in response to sun radiation which will lead to ugly and malignant changes. To start with, there may be drying or scaling and, as further time passes, cracks or fissures and whitish thickened areas may form on the lip or otherwise pigmented brown areas. These whitish areas may be called "leucoplakia" or "white patch". Sometimes such patches will form at the site of cigarette or pipe contact with the lip over a number of years. Leucoplakia can, in time, lead to a cancer of the lip.

Another lip change is the scaling or crusting often associated with a redness and irritability of the lip and this can be a "keratosis". With further years of sunshine this can progress, becoming a lip cancer. When either the keratosis or the leucoplakia start to become thickened, it is a sign that the cancer is starting to form and these things are better treated early when treatment is simple.

At times, a small pigmented or brown area will develop on the lip which may be similar to a dark freckle. This may enlarge which causes concern as it looks like it may grow to become a melanoma. They are often removed. In fact these pigmented spots on the lip are usually a benign "lentigo" and it is very rare for them to become a melanoma, but they are frequently unsightly and, with these pigmented spots, one cannot be sure just what they are until their microscopic pattern has been analysed. It is frequently more simple to have them removed and examined by the pathologist to be sure they are not a problem.

AVOIDING LIP DAMAGE

HATS

If you look at the hats that most people wear when they are out in the sun, you will see that the brim of the hat most often does not keep the sun off the lip. The eyes and the nose will be shaded but not the lip. Usually people are unaware of this. So, it is wise to wear an even broader brim to protect your lips and lower face. Most hats with broader brims are not well-ventilated and tend to keep a pocket of hot air underneath the brim. Most people wearing hats are most concerned with the fashion of the hat and generally hats with very broad brims are somewhat cumbersome and often unfashionable. So, some extra precaution is needed to protect the lips during time in the sun.

LIPSTICKS

Sunfilter lipsticks (such as Hamilton's Sola stick or Piz Buin lip and nose protector) have been formulated both to protect the lips from the drying effects of wind and heat and, in addition, to filter out ultraviolet radiation. The usual sunfilter can be put on the skin of the lips and then the sunfilter lipstick is applied.

The best opaque sun block lipsticks are the zinc ointments which form a thick coloured barrier against the ultraviolet with a protective effect that can last all day. It tends to be rather conspicuous and many people prefer to wear the translucent sunfilter lipstick, but the latter needs to be applied every two hours as it wears off.

CHANGES TO THE LIPS

If you are concerned about a spot on your lip, you should consult your doctor who will advise you what should be done and whether or not there is cause for concern. At times, a spot may simply need observation and may only need treatment if it continues to change. With early sun spots, a reduction in sun exposure and protection of that spot from the sun will often result in a reversal or a slowing of its development so that no further active treatment may be needed at that stage.

LIP CANCER

On the other hand, sometimes a small spot may require treatment and this can entail freezing (cryotherapy). Sometimes, the best treatment of a small early lesion is to cut it out under local anaesthetic and have the spot examined to determine whether it is malignant. It is important that the lip should be repaired well to give it a fine scar and an attractive normal contour. Depending on what is involved, your doctor may refer you to a specialist to have this done.

Larger lip lesions or sores may need to be cut out under anaesthetic with a wider margin of tissue, depending on the type of cancer involved. This is a specialised procedure which will often involve an initial biopsy, or examination of a small piece of the lump to confirm its nature, followed by excision to remove the dangerous part and then reconstructing the lip with appropriate tissue to produce the best looking and most functional result.

More advanced lip cancers may tend to spread to the lymph glands in the neck and these would need to be watched and removed if necessary. At times, an advanced cancer will have radiotherapy as well as surgery, or if the patient is not well enough for an operation, radiotherapy alone may be used. All of this can be avoided by early awareness of the possibility of cancer and avoidance of sun on the lip, particularly in childhood.

THE AGEING LIP

The fine contour of the lip margin and philtral columns cannot really be repaired by surgical means. But the vertical wrinkling of the skin above the upper lip, caused by the sun, can be treated by dermabrasion or chemical peeling. This treatment tends to cause a thinning of the skin and there can be secondary pigmentary problems. In general, the loss of lip elasticity is impossible to repair.

OTHER EFFECTS OF THE SUN ON THE LIP

People who tend to get cold sores (herpes) on the lip note that they will often get an attack of herpes after they have had a heavy dose of sun on the lip. We do know that ultraviolet radiation does reduce the immune system's ability to fight back. Ultraviolet does this by inhibiting some important cells in the skin which are normally responsible for holding infections, such as a herpes virus, in check. It is interesting that continued ultraviolet also reduces the ability of these same cells to deal with early cancer cells. Keeping the lip out of the sun will give the body's own immune system a much better chance of dealing with early sun spots.

CHAPTER 7

Moles, Sun Spots and Skin Cancers

Most people have brown marks on their skin of one sort or another. Mostly these are of no concern but sometimes they can be dangerous. How do we tell the difference between moles and sun spots and when can these be cancerous? If in doubt, any mark on the skin is best checked by your doctor.

FRECKLES

Freckles are brown spots on the fair-skinned, sun-sensitive people who have had sun exposure. They indicate the skin's inability to pigment evenly and are a sign of a sun-sensitive skin, resulting from over-stimulation of melanocytes (the pigment cells). To those who have them, they are the body's way of warning that it cannot cope with the sun; it is prone to skin cancer and premature ageing from sun damage. At times, instead of forming brown spots, the body will form white spots, the so-called "white freckles" which are a sign of exhaustion of the pigment cells from over-stimulation. If the skin is protected from the sun, such freckles will tend to go away in time.

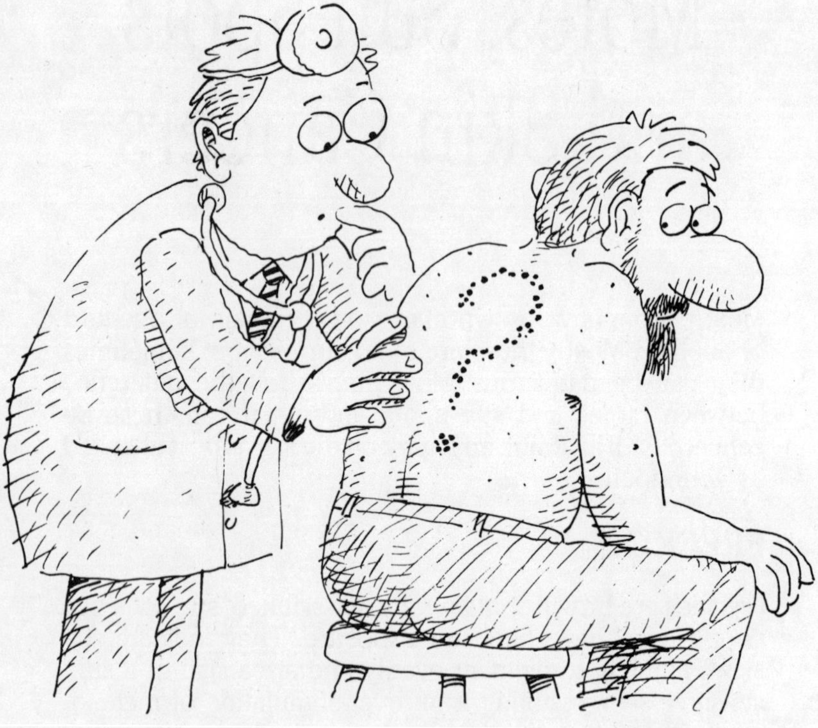

MOLES

Brown moles may be present at birth or they may come later as acquired moles or acquired naevi. Congenital naevi (pigmented) are the ones which are present at birth and these can be quite large. There is another type of non-pigmented or pale mole which can also be present.

Acquired naevi tend to form as a result of stimulation of the skin pigment cells by ultraviolet radiation and, with continued stimulation over the years, these may progress in their type and go on to form so-called dysplastic naevi. Continued ultraviolet stimulation on dysplastic naevi can sometimes result in the formation of melanomas.

It appears that short, sharp bursts of exposure to the sun on unprotected fair skin is most likely to cause change in moles and the production of melanomas. Most people who have developed melanomas have a history of attacks of sunburn some years previously. They are usually the more fair-skinned people, often the urban dweller who likes to pick up a quick tan at the weekend or in the holidays.

There are many innocent moles which are called benign naevi and these are often lighter brown in colour. They usually have a regular outline and their border is clearly defined. The average young adult will have about twenty-five brown moles and it is a good idea for those people who like to go out in the sun to become acquainted with their moles and know what they look like. This often involves the use of one or two mirrors and if there is a family history of melanoma, keeping photographs of your moles is a good way to remember what they were like.

It has been shown that, as the number of moles that a person has increases in number, so also does the chance of one of them changing and becoming dangerous, that is, becoming dysplastic or melanomatous.

SUSPICIOUS MOLES

The lighter brown moles which are raised, grow hairs and have a uniform colour are generally quite innocent. The flatter, darker, non-hairy moles can be a cause for concern, particularly if they have become darker.

An increase in the size of a mole can be cause for concern. In the case of growing children, the mole should only grow at the same rate as the rest of the child. Also with children, the moles generally do not become malignant before puberty but there have been rare cases where melanomas have developed in childhood. With darker or lumpier moles, care needs to be taken with observation of the mole and sometimes removal if it is considered to be dangerous.

Any change in the mole excites suspicion that it may be becoming dangerous. This can be change in colour, in size, in outline (from an even-rounded to an uneven outline) or in surface texture, perhaps with some irregularity. Change in colour of the mole such as the development of a lighter colour area or a darker colour area can excite suspicion of cellular activity and would warrant a visit to your doctor.

Moles that cause most concern have a variation in outline, surface texture and colour. There may be red, pale areas or bluish-black areas in the mole suggesting it is dangerous. Most moles do not have any feeling associated with them. When a feeling of itchiness develops or a feeling of unease abut the mole or a tingling sensation or bleeding or weeping from the mole then this can be a danger sign. It can be difficult to decide which moles should be removed and regular visits to check with your doctor may be worthwhile if you or your family are worried.

ACTION FOR SUSPICIOUS MOLES

When a mole has changed and is causing concern, it is better removed and examined under the microscope. In general, moles are removed completely and the whole mole examined. Good results are achieved in the treatment of melanoma by the early removal of suspicious moles so that the melanomas are then removed in the early phase of their development.

Melanomas actually go through stages of development

and in their early stages they are quite curable by a complete surgical removal. When present for a longer time, they go through different phases of development from the so-called horizontal phase to the so-called vertical phase and then become a more serious tumour, able to spread to other parts of the body, with unfortunate consequences.

DYSPLASTIC NAEVI

These are a particular kind of brown mole usually larger than the average small mole, often measuring some 7 to 11 mm. They tend to be varied in colour with darker and lighter spots, some pink areas perhaps and an uneven surface and outline. They can occur singly and may be the result of continued ultraviolet stimulation of other naevi and they are better removed.

Sometimes they can run in families where there are likely to be some who have had melanomas. People who have this so-called familial dysplastic naevus condition need to have their moles kept under regular medical observation and any suspicious ones removed.

SUN SPOTS

One of the early effects of ultraviolet radiation on the skin is a thickening of the outer horny layer which results from multiplication of the cells of the epidermis, and this thickening of the outer layer is in itself an extra filter. With continued ultraviolet radiation over the years, areas of overgrowth of the epidermis develop with the formation of thickened scaly patches called keratoses.

KERATOSES

Keratoses occur in sun-exposed regions such as the face, neck, forearm, back of the hand and other areas. They are typically scaly patches. Early keratoses may be reddened from dilated, small blood vessels in the skin and they may have a yellowish or brownish adherent scale or crust which may bleed when the crust is removed. At this stage of development, these changes can be halted or even reversed by keeping your skin out of the sun and protecting it from further exposure as this allows some repair to take place. The body's own immune system then has a chance to work uninhibited by the ultraviolet radiation. The surface scale can be reduced by a salicylic acid ointment and these may be sold in chemists as sun spot creams.

With continued ultraviolet exposure, the keratosis goes on to become larger and thicker. Later it starts to develop a fleshy thickening beneath. This is a sign of the early development of a squamous cell carcinoma or skin cancer, and at that stage it will need to be treated. Keratoses may be treated in the earlier stages and medical advice is desirable to make sure a more dangerous sun spot is not being mistaken for a simple one.

Earlier stages may be treated with an ointment such as 5-fluorouracil (Effudex). Freezing with liquid nitrogen (cryotherapy) is another method employed by many doctors. A shave excision under local anaesthetic (with microscopic examination) can also be used. Both the liquid nitrogen and the shave excision can leave pale areas when the treatment is extended through the layer of pigment-forming cells.

Early sun spots tend to come and go as they progress. When one is out in the sun and the skin is sheltered, they will tend to go away or become less obvious. This can be confusing as people think that there is a good chance that they will get better by themselves. In fact, early sun spots kept strictly out of the sun may not actually cure themselves but will certainly stop progressing.

LENTIGINES

These are flat brown spots rather like freckles but darker and they tend to occur in older people, although these days we find they are occurring in younger people because of their increased sun exposure. The fact that they are a brown spot can sometimes cause worry and they may occur on the back of the hand as well as on other sun-exposed parts of the body. They are frequently not dangerous and can at times be treated by simple methods. Bleaching ointments have been used. Shaving them off and sending to a pathologist establishes what they are and differentiates from the more dangerous pigmented spots. Bleaching ointments are based on a hydroxyquinone 2 per cent and a sunfilter to prevent further ultraviolet browning of the skin. They are best used under skilled supervision.

SENILE WARTS

These are the so-called seborrhoeic keratoses and they used to occur mainly in older people but now occur in younger people as well, some even in their thirties. They tend to be a darker, often greasy, raised, sometimes warty growth on the skin. They are unsightly and can be most simply treated by shaving them off under local anaesthetic, when, at that stage, their nature can be determined by a microscopic examination. They can also be treated by freezing with liquid nitrogen when the diagnosis is certain. They are not dangerous but can be confused with dangerous dark spots and for that reason they cause concern.

More serious skin cancers may also develop and there are a great variety of these. With experience, their nature may often be recognised from their appearance.

BASAL CELL CARCINOMA (RODENT ULCER)

The basal cell carcinoma (BCC) may have a great variety of different appearances. At times they may have a reddened crusty look somewhat similar to the keratosis, or they may simply have a red area on the skin with a slightly scaling surface. These are the superficial type of basal cell carcinomas.

On the other hand, a BCC may present as a lump, often with a pearly look to it when the skin is tightened. Sometimes there is only one of these or a few may develop close to each other. With time they enlarge. They may then tend to develop an ulcer in the centre, often with some lump or thickening. There is no pain or discomfort associated with this and the original description of this condition (the rodent ulcer) which came from Ireland in 1827 was of an ulcer of the face which had been present for many years quietly eating away at the tissues. This was the reason for the original term "rodent ulcer".

At other times, the BCC may be quite inconspicuous, perhaps just a slightly puckered or scaling area but with a deeper thickening beneath and a tendency to invade — the so-called infiltrating BCC.

At other times, the BCC may simply be a whitish plaque in the skin, quite inconspicuous and perhaps not noticed for some years. Recognising the BCC, which type it is and its appropriate treatment, whether it be surgery or cryotherapy (freezing with liquid nitrogen), is the work of an expert and your doctor should be consulted. Radiotherapy, these days, is usually reserved for older people or for those unfit for other methods of treatment, because of the long-term damaging effect of the radiation on the tissues that are left behind.

Basal cell carcinomas remain limited to the one area of the body where they have originated and do not tend to spread to other parts. Properly treated, with complete removal, they should cause no further trouble although the area needs to be kept under observation for some years, partly to make sure they do not recur, and partly to identify any new tumours that may develop in that same area.

SQUAMOUS CELL CARCINOMA

One further skin cancer type which may develop in those with long sun exposure is the squamous cell carcinoma

(SCC). These also have a variety of appearances. They may be a crusted area which, with time, has become thickened. Initially, perhaps it was a solar keratosis which, after being present for quite a long period, became thickened beneath and was then an early phase of squamous cell carcinoma. These are usually slow-growing initially and do *not* tend to spread to other parts of the body.

There is a second type of squamous cell carcinoma which tends to develop as a more fleshy nodule. This is more rapid-growing and often tends to spread — in time to other parts of the body. Sometimes a benign condition called a keratoacanthoma may also be fleshy and rapid-growing. It tends to fall off in a period of three to four months but there may be confusion in identifying the lump. Medical opinion is advised with removal and examination of the lump. Generally, there are other signs of sun damage with loss of elastic tissue, irregular pigmentation and scaly patches occurring around squamous cell carcinomas and basal cell carcinomas.

The treatment of squamous cell carcinoma is generally that it should be excised (cut out) with a margin of normal tissue and the resulting hole or defect is closed by bringing in fresh tissue in a reconstructive operation designed to result in minimum scarring or distortion.

At times, with the rapid-growing, aggressive, squamous cell carcinoma, radiotherapy will be used as well as surgery to control the cancer. This type can spread to the regional lymphatic glands in the neck, groin, or armpit and these sites need to be kept under observation. If the glands become enlarged they may require surgical removal.

Once again, it is better to treat this SCC condition at an earlier biological stage before it has become advanced and aggressive. That is to say, it is better to have suspicious areas looked at in the early stages.

MALIGNANT MELANOMAS

Pigmented spots have received much publicity in recent

years because of the risk that they may become a malignant melanoma. This is usually the darker-coloured tumour which develops from a mole. It can often be dark brown, sometimes even approaching black. While most melanomas are pigmented, there are also types of melanoma which do not have the dark colour and this makes them harder to recognise but the microscopic pattern can be detected and there are special stains which reveal to the pathologist the type of tumour with which he is dealing. Melanomas need to be removed more widely although this will depend on the phase of development they have reached.

There are three phases in melanoma development. The first is the slow growing, flat, lentigo maligna melanoma. Here, there is a blotchy irregular pigmentation (colour) and irregular outline with darker and lighter areas and sometimes a little thickening.

A later stage is the superficial spreading melanoma. This may be a slightly elevated and perhaps a brown-crusting lesion with a poorly defined edge and sometimes some red areas associated. With a further passage of time, sometimes years, the melanoma may then go from the initial horizontal phase into the vertical phase in which case it becomes more thickened or lumpy and sometimes will develop an ulcer or sore, perhaps with some bleeding or oozing of serum.

At times, any of these different phases of melanoma may develop what is called regression in which there may be a hollowing of contour and perhaps a loss of pigment producing a lighter colour where the tumour has been attacked by the body's defence mechanism (the immune system) causing part of it to regress. The fact that areas of regression have occurred doesn't mean that the body is able to overcome the tumour. This may happen at times, but is not to be relied upon, especially with melanomas.

The treatment of melanomas is surgical removal and treatment at the early stage is more effective. Treatment of the later stages also is well worthwhile but more complicated involving removal of the melanoma and perhaps the regional lymph glands if they become involved or perhaps other areas as well. Melanoma can often be quite slow-growing and unpredictable and it is worth treating it even in advanced stages.

The emphatic point in the treatment of melanoma is that in the early stages it is a very curable disease. It has been shown by the Queensland Melanoma Project that the best results in the world can be achieved by treatment of the early phase, educating people to come and seek expert advice with the early change in moles and pigmented spots so that the disease is removed before the more advanced phase develops.

THE BODY'S IMMUNE RESPONSE

Ultraviolet radiation passing through the skin into the cells of the epidermis causes a change in the DNA, the compound that controls the activity of the cell. These DNA changes then are likely to result in abnormal behaviour of the cell which, in time, leads to further change resulting in malignancy. There is a repair process in the body mediated by a specific enzyme group which enables removal of the damaged DNA. There is a rare familial disease in which this enzyme is lacking and these people tend to have a specific tendency to form skin cancers. (This disease is called Xeroderma Pigmentosum.)

Normally, the immune system of one's body will identify cells with damaged DNA and try to dispose of them. Ultraviolet light, however, damages those cells responsible for mediating the immune response, and, in particular, the Langerhans cells which are normally found in the epidermis.

It has been found that, with chronic sun exposure, Langerhans cell population numbers decrease quite dramatically, and this also happens with age. In addition, radiation of the Langerhans cells with Ultraviolet-B destroys their ability to act and to point out the damaged cells to the immune system.

It has been shown that a specific immune incompetence develops for sun-induced tumour cells because of further ultraviolet radiation from the sun.

We also know that the immune system is suppressed by drugs taken after kidney transplants to prevent rejection of the donor kidney, and those people, with subsequent sun exposure, have a very high incidence of skin cancers because of their immune incompetence.

Thus, we are able to say that, not only does ultraviolet radiation cause change in the DNA to produce skin cancers, but it also inhibits the immune response that would normally help to get rid of these damaged cells. The importance of this knowledge lies in the fact that it is worth keeping your skin out of the sun to help in the repair of the damaged cells. *It is never too late to start taking precautions* because there will be benefits even at a later age from keeping your skin out of the sun.

CHAPTER 8

Caring for Your Skin

Skin care is important for both children and adults. Even though good habits are best begun in childhood, it is never too late to be kind to your skin.

SKIN APPEARANCE

The natural beauty of the skin is achieved first of all by having an elastic skin which has a supple contour and clothes the body elegantly without folds or creases. It is also achieved by the appearance of the skin surface which is most attractive when smooth and even and having a lustre or "bloom". A good moisture content in the skin is one of the important things for this surface appearance. How is all of this affected by the sun?

MOISTURE CONTENT

One of the earlier effects of sun exposure is to cause a thickening of the outer horny or squamous layer of the skin, causing it to dry out and lose moisture. At this stage the application of creams and ointments to return moisture to the outer layer of the skin is important. People living in very hot climates observe that their skin will absorb

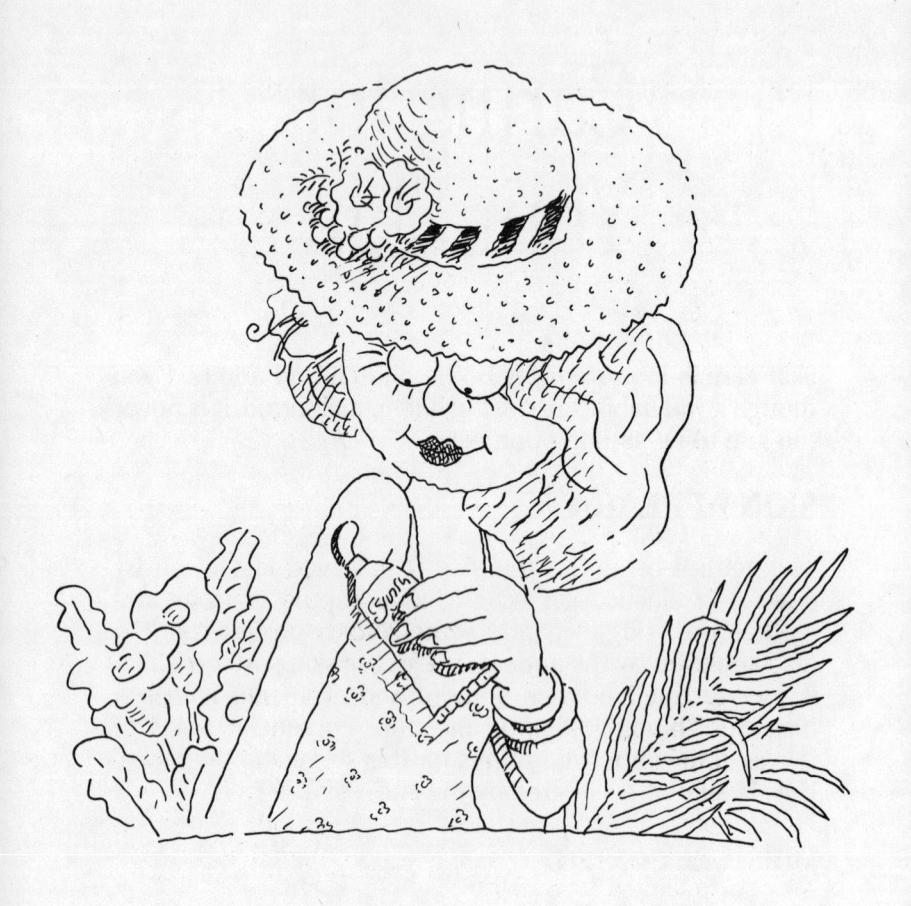

much more cream especially in drier, windier areas. Thickening of the outer skin does improve the skin's sun resistance but it worsens its appearance.

WRINKLES

Early skin wrinkling can appear between the age of 20 and 35 years. This is due to the ultraviolet radiation penetrating into the skin and not only causing drying and reduction of moisture, but also relaxation of elasticity. This results from loss of the elastin fibres, in particular, but also of the collagen. Some things will tend to accentuate this, for example, cigarette smoking reduces the nutrition of the skin, while Vitamin C does tend to have some protective effect.

The skin must be elastic so that it can expand and contract with movement, breathing, eating or just becoming fat and thin again. In order to be elastic, the skin has a deeper layer called *the dermis*. In the dermis, run networks of coiled springy fibres called elastin and collagen. Collagen has a strong coil structure and is manufactured and maintained by cells called fibroblasts. Elastin fibres are more springy and rubbery. These fibres sit in a jelly-like "ground" substance which forms the foundation of the skin texture.

The *surface of the skin* is formed by the epidermis and this has an outer layer of cells which are flattened or "squamous". These cells are produced in the epidermis and layers of them are constantly being formed to act as its outer protective cover. This outer horny layer is constantly being rubbed off. If it is removed too much, the cell layer beneath may be injured.

BLEMISHES

A blotchy discolouration can be an early sign of sun damage in some younger people. This is associated with dryness of the skin and some thickening of the outer layer.

SKIN ASSISTANCE

When you realise that your skin is ageing more quickly than you wish, begin to take more care with sun exposure and use the sunfiltering and protective measures described elsewhere in this book. Additional methods are outlined below.

OINTMENTS

It is important to return moisture to the skin and to keep the skin well lubricated and supple. Moisturising creams or oils can be selected to suit your skin. The better moisturising creams will often have a sunfilter built into them. Good advice can be obtained from either beauty consultants or cosmetic counters in well-known stores regarding the best type of creams, lotions, oils or ointments for your skin. These will improve the moisture in the skin and its appearance.

SYNTHETIC VITAMIN A OINTMENTS

If your skin has suffered damage to its structure, there are hopes that the use of the so-called retinoids (Retin A) ointments in the long term will help to restore the skin to what it was prior to sun damage or to maintain it without further deterioration. These ointments only work when one is avoiding further ultraviolet exposure and indeed one must do that when using them as they are photosensitisers and will increase the damaging action of sunlight on the skin. They will irritate some skins and there is some exfoliative action associated with them so that some initial redness of the skin may result. It is better to start with a lower concentration of ointment and slowly increase this and it is also better to initially only apply the ointment at night a couple of times a week and then to steadily build up to a once or twice daily use. Those who promote these ointments believe that their prolonged use will result in a retention of a more youthful skin. Medical advice is desirable when using these products.

OTHER REPAIR CREAMS

Other creams are also sold whose promoters believe that they will help to repair the damaged fibrous and cellular structures in the skin with long-term usage and avoidance of ultraviolet. We will need to wait a number of years before we see the long-term effects of these ointments and it may well be that the general care of the skin associated with their use and avoidance of sunlight in damaging amounts will help produce a better quality of skin.

WASHING PROCEDURES

It pays to remember that soaps and detergents remove oils from the skin and that soaps vary in their severity. In attempting to keep as much oil in the skin as possible it is wise to limit the use of soap on the skin to that which is essential and to make a practice of replacing oil and moisture that has been removed from the skin.

SKIN PEELING

Skin peeling is said to improve the skin by stimulating growth of the epidermal and connective tissue cells. This can be in the form of a paste which is spread onto the skin for some fifteen to twenty minutes and then scraped off. These are often resorcinol-based ointments or "unnas paste" type ointments. This procedure leaves the skin red for the first two days, with a slight brownish tinge on the third day, the skin peeling on the fourth, fifth and sixth days. Absolute avoidance of the sun is necessary during this time. This type of skin peeling is used for early wrinkling and skin thickening and, combined with good skin care, will help in the early stages. Later on, when the wrinkling becomes deeper and more intense, a chemical skin peel can be used. These treatments require careful supervision from an experienced practitioner.

For a chemical skin peel, a mixture of phenol, soap and croton oil is applied to the skin as a specific layer with great care taken to achieve an even application and to avoid eyes, mouth and so on. Careful medical supervision is necessary. This treatment, in effect, produces a chemical burn of the skin which results in loss of the surface with redness, irritation and pain, and the necessity to prevent infection by the use of anti-bacterial ointments or powders. The surface usually takes two weeks or so to heal depending on the depth of the burn. It will smooth out surface wrinkles and the effect at first is of a red uniform skin which must be kept out of the sun for the first three months or so. Sometimes there is a loss of the normal colouring in the skin when the epidermal cells responsible for normal pigmentation have been destroyed by the burn. At other times, if one goes out in the sun too early, a blotchy pigmentation can result. For this reason people having chemical peels of this type need to be prepared to wear make-up, possibly for the rest of their lives, as the pigmentation changes are unpredictable. Some people are less likely to have pigmentary problems and other people more likely, depending on their skin type.

COLLAGEN TREATMENT

With this treatment there is an attempt to remove the wrinkles by injecting an animal collagen derivative into the dermis, just below the epidermis of the skin to fill out the grooves. Different types of collagen are available on the market but they are all animal products and each individual needs to be sensitivity-tested before having this treatment. Certainly, the collagen can fill out contour defects in the skin surface but the problem is that the effect lasts only a few months. In some people effects last as little as one month but in others, it may last up to twelve months. People having treatment of fine surface wrinkling by collagen must be prepared to attend repeatedly for as long as they want the effect to be maintained. The wrinkling around the mouth which seems to worry people quite a lot is subject to movement of the mouth and this seems to cause an early resorption of much of the injectable collagen. At other times allergic responses may be encountered as the repeated injection of foreign protein is one of the ways to sensitise people to that protein and the allergic response can result in red lumps which may require steroids to settle them down.

AGEING SKIN

With further ageing of the skin, there is not only a loss of elastic tissue but the surface of the skin itself seems to expand so that there is more loose tissue in folds on the back of the hands, the face, the neck, the eyelids, and so on, really in all the areas of the body that are affected by the ultraviolet radiation. This looseness of the skin also causes a drop of the cheeks, a drop of the neck and a drop of the eyelids. What has not been realised by many people who engage in topless bathing, is that the skin of the breast exposed to the sun will also expand and lose its elastic tissue, causing the breasts to drop. Once the cheeks and neck have dropped in this way, ointments or chemical peels are not going to bring them back.

FACELIFT

The technique of lifting the skin of the face, tightening the deeper muscles and lifting up the cheeks and neck is known as a facelift. These surgical procedures have developed since their beginning in the early 1900s when they were really only a skinlift. Since that time the techniques of lifting the facial planes and muscles to restore facial contour as well as removal of fat to enhance the contour of the neck and parts of the cheeks has developed and there are now a number of different facelifts which can be applied to the needs of the patient.

Eyelids: Excess skin in the eyelids can be removed putting scars into the crease lines of the eyelid, removing or relocating fat deposits, and, depending on the need, the muscular dynamic contour of the eyelid can be realigned.

It must be borne in mind, however, that these surgical procedures do not return elasticity to the skin; they simply tighten and lift the skin and they need to be taken in conjunction with other measures to improve the skin itself and to arrest the damage from further ultraviolet radiation.

Lip Wrinkling: Wrinkling of the upper lip can be a problem in the sun-damaged and, when this is deep, the best treatment is probably what is known as a dermabrasion in which the surface of the skin is sandpapered off by a sterile surgical device and the surface allowed to heal over the next seven to ten days. This procedure results in a marked improvement in the contour and loss of the deeper wrinkles. This surface again needs to be kept out of the sun for the first few months to avoid over-tanning. Dermabrasion can also result in a loss of some of the normal pigmentation and make-up may be needed.

Forehead: Wrinkling of the forehead can at times be improved by dermabrasion as with wrinkling of the lip but at other times a skinlift on the forehead and a relocation of the forehead muscle may be necessary in a procedure known as a browlift. This can also elevate the eyebrows which have dropped as a result of the lengthening of the sun-damaged forehead skin. The dropped eyebrow will push extra skin into the upper eyelid and also give an expression in which the person appears to be rather tired or disinterested or scowling. Elevation of the brow can improve not only the wrinkling of the forehead but also the expression and the appearance of the upper eyelid.

With these operations there is some loss of sensation

because of the necessity to divide small nerves to the skin in the operation. Most of this feeling will return.

CONCLUSION

Skin care is a wide-ranging subject, however, basic guidelines can be followed no matter how much skin damage has been sustained. It is important firstly to protect children's skin and secondly to prevent your own skin from suffering further damage.

The body's own immune system offers a mechanism for repair of sun damaged skin but cannot work effectively unless it is assisted by a healthy lifestyle, which should start with an avoidance of ultraviolet exposure. There are many other contributing factors.

- Regular exercise to stimulate blood circulation which in turn benefits the skin.
- A balanced diet which avoids excess animal fats and sugars, with a high fibre content and plenty of fresh vegetables and fruit.
- Avoidance of smoking as nicotine reduces skin circulation and in the long-term produces a dried out, sallow look.
- Excess alcohol is to be avoided as it damages the system generally. Alcohol is a neurotoxin (damages the nerves and the brain) and while it is a stimulant in small quantities, in large quantities, it is a depressant.
- Protective clothing is more economical and convenient than overall sunscreen cover, and can also look attractive.
- The use of vitamin supplements, in particular Vitamin C with its specific repair properties.
- Night creams on sensitive areas such as the face, neck and hands.
- Finally, drinking water is the great unsung stand-by of a healthy life. It should become a habit to have a glass of water in the morning and on the meal table, and especially when drinking wine.

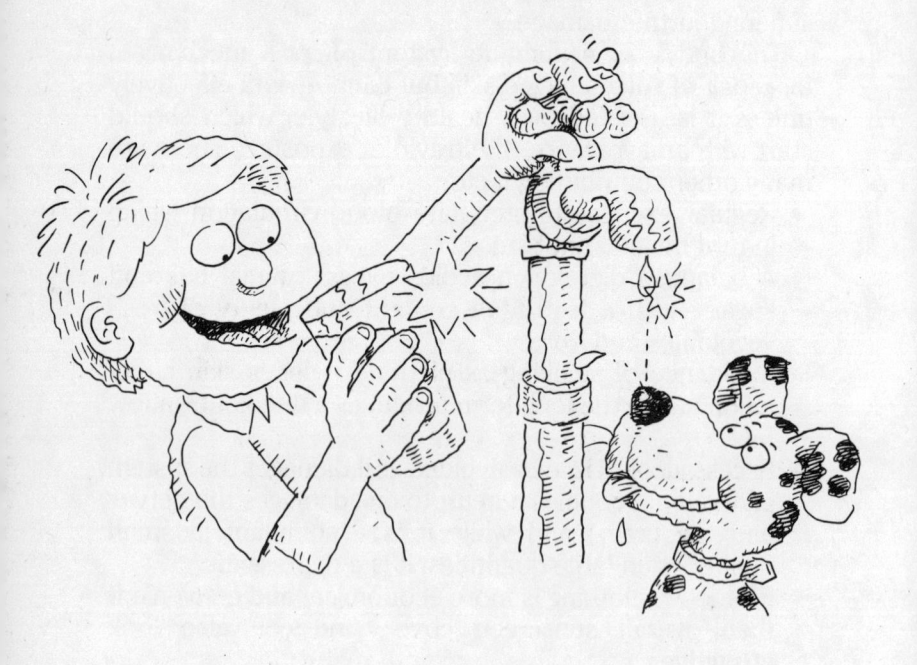

CHAPTER 9

Other Effects of Strong Sunshine

When we are in the sun, the body keeps itself cool by sweating or perspiring and this moisture on the skin surface evaporates, absorbing the latent heat of evaporation from the body and thus cooling it. As we work harder in the heat, this mechanism of cooling becomes important to our survival and takes priority over all other requirements for body water.

In the short term this does not matter very much but in the long term, if we are not drinking enough water, the body will still take what it needs for perspiration leaving the kidneys habitually short of water to excrete the by-products of the body's metabolism. We have no way of knowing that the body is short of water as the sense of thirst is not dependable. The only way to tell that the kidneys are having to concentrate the urine unduly because of a shortage of water is to see that the urine is more deeply coloured. Urine should naturally be only a light straw colour or very pale yellow. The kidneys have no way of telling us that we are not drinking enough water to allow for both perspiration and for kidney excretion. In the long term this shortage of water and over-concentration by the kidneys can lead not only to the formation of kidney stones but also to various kidney diseases.

PREVENTION OF KIDNEY DISEASE

People in cooler climates get used to not having to drink so much water because there isn't the need for a lot of perspiration passing through the skin. Drinking is actually habitual. Children growing up in the tropics or in hot climates need to be taught to drink one or two tumblers of water each morning before they do anything else. They also need to be taught to drink more water during the day when they are doing things out in the sun or working hard and producing a lot of perspiration.

Failure to provide the kidneys with adequate fluids over a number of years results in a high incidence of the formation of kidney stones. These kidney stones can injure the kidney and may be very painful when they are being passed. In the past, larger stones were removed by surgery but these days they can be broken up with a sonic shock machine. It is better, however, to avoid forming stones by keeping a better urine flow.

Various substances such as lead, tablets including phenacetin, and other substances may injure the kidney when the urine is heavily concentrated and kept in the kidneys because of a shortage of water in the system. Over the years, chronic injury to the kidney by water shortage can result in the need for a kidney transplant. Surgeons who are associated with patients having kidney transplants note that these patients need to learn to drink enough water to protect their new kidney.

In the hotter parts of Australia we have one of the world's highest incidences per head of population of both kidney stones and the need for kidney transplants.

BABIES

Remember that babies are much more prone to fluid loss than are adults so try to avoid any situation where the child is exposed to the loss of excessive water, as this will necessitate quite a lot of drinking. It is a good idea also to see that the baby is passing an adequate urine volume.

Avoid leaving babies in a hot car and try always to have sunshades for them. Those big sunshade canopies on strollers keep the baby cool and avoid sun exposure. They will still need some suncream for reflected ultraviolet on strong days, however. If you are out in the heat, carry extra water for your young children and yourself.

DEHYDRATION HEADACHES

A shortage of water can result in a headache. This type of dehydration headache was part of the effect previously known as "sunstroke". We must remember that, with a headache in hot weather, drinking two tumblers of water is as helpful as pain-relieving tables.

It is perhaps an irony that long-term damage to the kidneys associated with long-term body water shortage and the taking of certain painkilling tablets, can result in a rise of the blood pressure level and this, in itself, may produce more headache.

You can monitor your water intake by watching the colour of your urine and it is wise to drink enough water to keep your urine looking reasonably clear. A slight pale yellowing is alright but the colour shouldn't habitually be darker. This urine colour is your first indication of the need to drink more fluid.

HANGOVERS

Alcoholic beverages of all kinds tend to increase the flow of urine from the kidneys and so are called "diuretics". This, in itself, does no harm but if the body is already dehydrated from not drinking enough water, the consumption of a diuretic, useful though it is to flush out the kidneys, will result in the body being even more short of water afterwards. This shortage of water is one of the reasons for the headache associated with the hangover. The best way to avoid this is to drink two tumblers of water after the consumption of alcohol and before you go to bed and perhaps take some Vitamin B at the same time, as the alcohol must be "burnt" by the liver and the Vitamin B helps.

People living in hot climates often take some alcohol to help them sleep at night as sleeping in the heat can at times be difficult. They should compensate by drinking two tumblers of water in the morning.

CHAPTER 10

Living Without the Sun

Changing climatic conditions and the increase in skin cancer makes it imperative that we rethink our lifestyles.

Living as we do in an age in which the tan has held social prominence for so long, it takes some mental adjustment to decide to do without it. It is true that models and well-known people are starting to appear with white skins and it is starting to be recognised that the tan is not the healthy thing that it was once thought to be. Nevertheless, there are many steps to be taken in the decision to live avoiding major sun exposure. It is, in fact, a way of life.

MENTAL ATTITUDE

Once a conscious decision has been made that your skin is going to look better and last longer without the sun, you will need to develop certain mental resources to go with this attitude. So much of our advertising emphasises that attractive people have a tan, that most of our society believes this. In fact it is more attractive to avoid the sun and to highlight the natural skin colouring, its lustrous texture and supple elegance. Preserving the elastic tissue in the skin will also preserve the contour of your cheeks

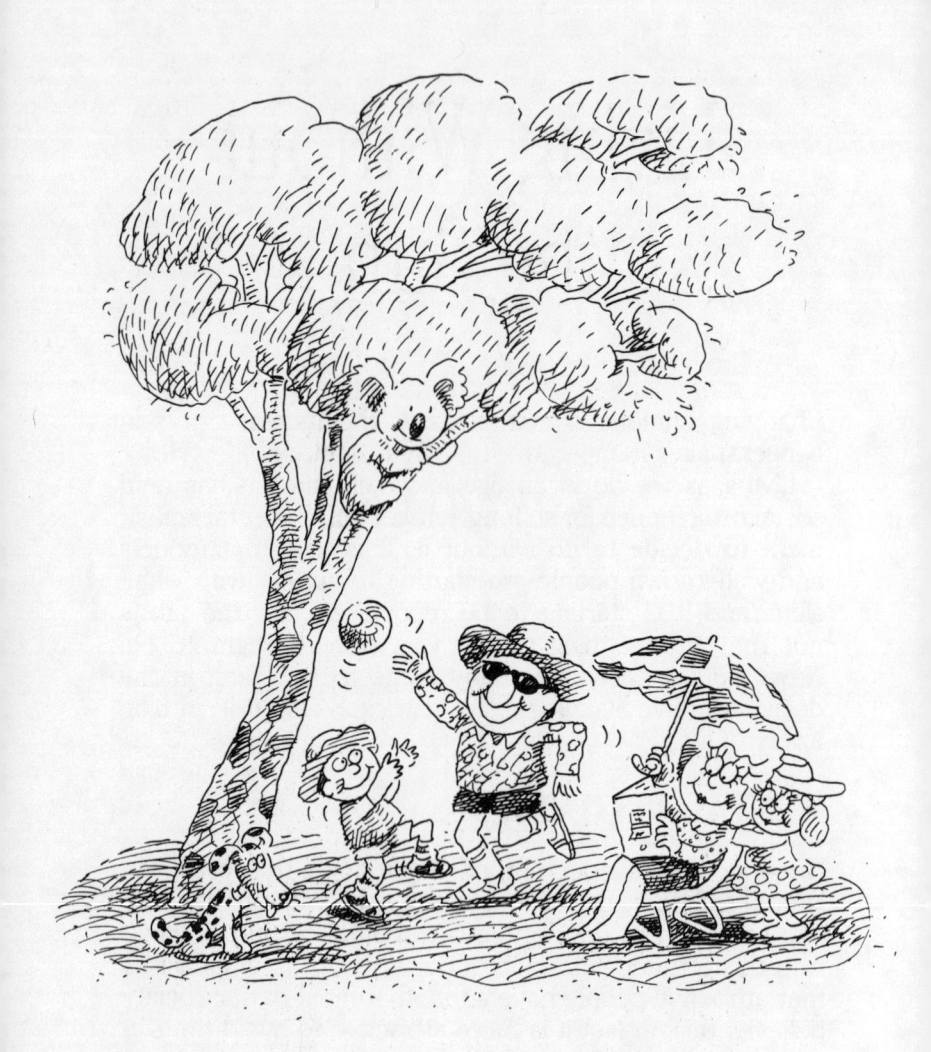

and neck, breasts and thighs. Much of the looseness of the thigh that comes to habitual suntanners is from loss of the elastic fibres in the skin and consequent flabbiness and wrinkling.

It is important that we believe our natural colouring is beautiful and do not constantly try to tan. It is unnatural for types I and II skins (see Chapter 2) to be tanned when nature has intended them to be fair.

It has been said that wealthy and famous people are never seen without a tan. There is this continued implication that if you can afford an elegant lifestyle, you will have a tan picked up at your villa by the sea, on your yacht, or if you live in a cold climate then you probably picked up the tan by flying to some tropical or sunny paradise where you keep your getaway home. Certainly, the measure of luxury has always been the vision of the sun-drenched life with all its accompanying luxuries. We must now recognise that this need not be so.

ADVERTISING

Even though the government and various cancer societies have advertised extensively about the dangers of the sun, there still remains a widespread desire for young people to be brown. Tourist areas in Australia, America, along the Mediterranean coast of Europe, the Pacific and New Zealand, show tourists arriving with fair skins, becoming bright red in the sun and going brown. In addition to being destructive to the beauty of the skin, this is also highly dangerous, causing the formation of melanomas, the most aggressive of skin cancers affecting young people. It is a tribute to the power of advertising that the attractiveness of brown skin in so many advertisements can push people into such painful, debilitating and dangerous activities as deliberate suntanning with an unsuitable skin. While it is true that not everybody has an unsuitable skin and those with skin types III and IV can tan quite well, they, too, will suffer the later effects of chronic sun exposure.

The skin is like a cocoon enveloping the body, the health of the skin is as important as the rest of the body. Care of the skin begins at birth. Parents need to be aware of the vulnerability of babies' and children's skin and take special care to avoid setting the stage for skin cancers later in life. Children in strollers should never be placed in direct sunlight — always provide shade. Protective clothing should be worn by both children and parents, and sunscreens used whenever necessary.

RECREATION

Recreation is an essential part of a healthy lifestyle and it is possible to reorganise activities taking the sun into account. In order to limit sun exposure, it is desirable to arrange outdoor games in the non-sunny periods of the day. Try to organise your golf in the early morning. Pressure tournament organisers to change their starting times accordingly. Tennis is another example. Playing tennis at night on a floodlit court is now relatively easy as such courts are readily available and not only is it safer but it is also much cooler, especially in summer.

In countries like Canada and North America, they usually put an inflatable "bubble" over the tennis court so that it can be used in winter as well as summer. The covering may also act as an ultraviolet filter, as it is a large polythene envelope held up by air pressure from a fan blowing in air.

With a little thought and planning, recreational activities can be safe from the effects of the sun.

Beaches are compelling but so too are forests. Beaches should be avoided during the middle of the day and you should always be aware of the dangers of reflected ultraviolet light even on cloudy days. Forests on the other hand absorb ultraviolet rays creating an environment much kinder to your skin.

Avoiding skin damage is a lifelong exercise involving every aspect of life. With a little thought and planning, our health can only benefit.

APPENDIX

The Structure of Light

We see things by visible light which is white light. White light is made up of a combination of colours — red, orange, yellow, green, blue, purple and violet, the so-called spectrum of light.

Visible light is simply one of the forms of energy which comes to us from the sun, and with it there is a whole range of different energy forms. The range of this energy is called the electromagnetic spectrum, and visible light lies in the middle of the range.

This energy comes in waves, like the waves of the ocean, and high energy radiation has a shorter distance between the waves, so that by measuring the wavelength (the distance between waves) we have an idea of the energy. Wavelengths are measured in billionths of a metre, or nanometres (nm). Thus, Ultraviolet-C has more energy than Ultraviolet-A and has a shorter wavelength.

VISIBLE LIGHT

Visible light lying in the centre of the spectrum of radiant energy has a wavelength between 400nm and 800nm. When light is passed through a prism, it is broken up into its constituent colours as described above, which is the effect one sees with the colours of the rainbow.

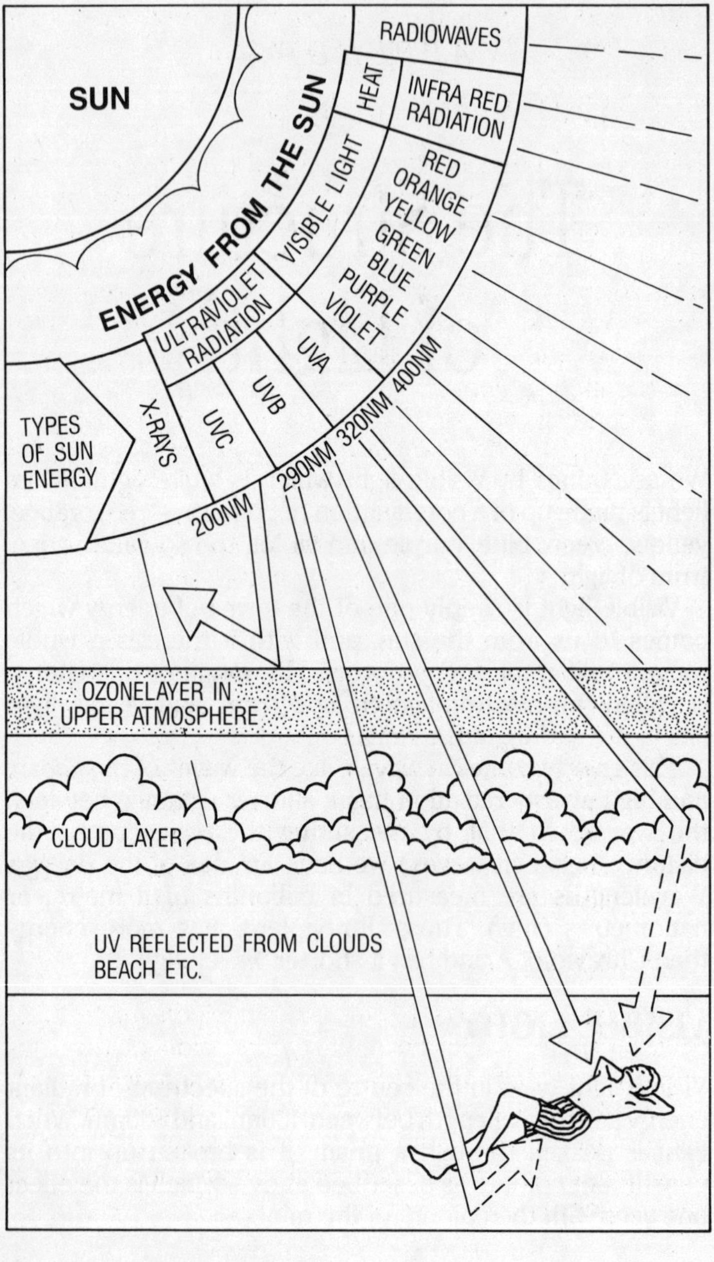
SUN
ENERGY FROM THE SUN
RADIOWAVES
HEAT
INFRA RED RADIATION
VISIBLE LIGHT
RED
ORANGE
YELLOW
GREEN
BLUE
PURPLE
VIOLET
ULTRAVIOLET RADIATION
UVA
UVB
UVC
X-RAYS
TYPES OF SUN ENERGY
200NM
290NM
320NM
400NM
OZONELAYER IN UPPER ATMOSPHERE
CLOUD LAYER
UV REFLECTED FROM CLOUDS BEACH ETC.

Infra-red energy lying above 800nm is not visible nor is ultraviolet radiation lying below 400nm.

ULTRAVIOLET RADIATION

This form of radiant energy is considered to have three different types — Ultraviolet-A (UV-A) has the lower energy (400–320nm), next comes Ultraviolet-B (UV-B) (320–290nm) and finally Ultraviolet-C (UV-C) the highest energy (290–200nm). X-rays are the next form of radiant energy with a wavelength below 200nm indicating more energy again than the Ultraviolet-C (UV-C). More energy again is found in the gamma rays.

We can see then that Ultraviolet-C (UV-C) radiation is almost as powerful as X-rays. Fortunately, it is reflected or filtered out by the ozone layer so that up until now Ultraviolet-C (UV-C) has not been reaching the surface of the Earth. Ultraviolet-B (UV-B) is the main ultraviolet which affects us and it is the one that is known to cause skin cancers and ageing of the skin.

For a long time Ultraviolet-A (UV-A) was thought to be relatively harmless but we now know that it will penetrate deeply into the dermis of the skin causing degeneration of the elastic and collagen fibres which make up the strength and structure of the dermis, the backing of the skin which gives it its supple strength and texture. Ultraviolet-A (UV-A) is now also known to predispose us to the effects of Ultraviolet-B (UV-B) in causing changes in the cells of the skin that lead to skin cancers.

MIDDAY ULTRAVIOLET

Ultraviolet is more dangerous in the middle of the day because there is a more direct penetration of the rays of the sun at that time. This is when the sun lies directly overhead and there is less of the Earth's atmosphere for the rays to pass through before getting to us. In this way, there is less of it absorbed and so it becomes more powerful and dangerous.

ULTRAVIOLET TRANSMISSION

On a cloudy day much of the light from the sun is absorbed in the cloud layer as is much of the infra-red radiation which causes the heat. Quite a lot of the ultraviolet radiation is also absorbed but still much of it gets through.

It helps to remember that ultraviolet radiation is somewhat like X-rays that penetrate. Similarly, ultraviolet radiation can penetrate into the skin and it does not stop at the surface. Ultraviolet-A (UV-A) penetrates into the mid-dermis affecting the fibres of the skin, causing them to age and Ultraviolet-B (UV-B) penetrates through the stratum corneum, the outer horny layer, to affect the living skin cells and the fibres.

Ultraviolet-A (UV-A) has been used in solariums generated by sunlamps and were once thought to be safe but it is now realised that it is not safe and causes ageing of the skin and also a predisposition to skin cancer. Ultraviolet-A (UV-A) is able to pass through the glass of the motorcar whereas Ultraviolet-B (UV-B) is mostly absorbed by the motorcar windscreen or windows. The extent of transmission will vary with the type of glass. Terylene foil is an excellent Ultraviolet-B (UV-B) absorber but polythene foil transmits more than 50 per cent of Ultraviolet-B (UV-B).

INDEX

Ageing of skin, 39, 45, 66, 69, 83
   premature, 7
   see also Skin damage
Alcohol, 71, 75–76
Antihistamines, 37
Appearance *see* Physical
   appearance

Babies
   dehydration, danger of, 74–75
   skin damage of, 13, 33
   skin protection for, 33–34, 75, 80
   see also Children
Basal cell carcinoma, 57–58
Beaches *see* Lifestyle; Swimming
Blemishes, 65
Burn time, 18, 28, 35, 40

Cancer, 7, 51–62
   treatment *see* Surgical
   remedies
   see also Basal cell carcinoma;
   Keratoses; Lentigines; Lips;
   Melanoma; Moles; Squamous
   cell carcinoma; Sun spots
Cars *see* Motorcars
Children
   lips, 46, 49
   skin damage of, 13, 33
   skin protection for, 33, 80
   see also Babies
Clothing
   as sun protection, 23–26, 71, 80
Collagen, 45, 65, 68
   see also Skin damage, repair of
Cosmetics *see* Make-up

Creams, 30, 48–49, 63, 66–67, 71
   see also Moisturisers
Damage to skin *see* Skin damage
Dark skin *see* Skin types
Dehydration, 74–75
Dermabrasion *see* Peeling,
   chemical peel
Diet
   and skin care, 71
Dyplastic naevi *see* Moles

Ears
   protection of, 25
Elasticity of skin, 44, 47, 49, 63,
   65, 69, 70, 77–79
Employment
   exposure to sun during, 20
Environment, 9, 32–33
   see also Lifestyle
Exercise, 71
   see also Sport
Eye
   effects of sun on, 41–44

Facelift, 69–71
Fair skin *see* Skin Types
Freckles, 17, 38, 51

Gloves, 25
Greenhouse effect, 11

Hats, 25–26, 47–48
Health
   association with tan, 12, 14, 19, 77
   skin care and, 71
   see also Lifestyle

Herpes, 50

Immune system, 38, 50, 61–62, 71
see also Ultraviolet radiation, effect on immune system of; Langerhans cells

Keratoses, 25, 55–56
Kidney disease, 73–74

Langerhans cells, 38, 60–61
Layers of the skin, 15
Lentigines, 56–57
Lifestyle, 7, 9, 11, 32, 71, 77–80
Lips, 45–50
  cancer of, 47, 49
  damage to, 48–49, 50, 70
Lipsticks
  as sun protection, 48
  see also Make-up

Make-up, 27, 31–32
  see also Lipsticks
Melanin see Pigmentation
Melanoma, 38, 47, 53, 59–61
Moisturisers, 63–67
  see also Creams
Moles, 53–55
  ultraviolet stimulation of, 53
Motorcars, 25, 34, 75, 84

Olive skin see Skin types
Ozone layer, 7, 10

Parasols see Umbrellas
Peeling
  chemical peel, 49, 67–68, 70
Photosensitivity, 38–39, 51, 66
  see also Skin types; Sunscreens, sensitivity to
Physical appearance, 12, 63, 77–79
  see also Tan
Pigmentation, 15, 17, 19, 21–22, 26, 31, 38, 51, 68

Protection from sun see Sun protection methods

Recreation see Lifestyle
Reflected rays, 20, 25, 35, 44, 75, 80
Retinoid derivatives, 39, 66
  see also Ageing and skin; Skin damage, repair of

Sensitive skin see Photosensitivity
Skin
  reaction to sunscreens see Sunscreens, sensitivity to
Skin cancer see Cancer
Skin care, 20–21, 31–32, 63–71
  see also Creams; Make-up; Moisturisers; Sunscreens
Skin damage, 12–14, 51
  repair of, 39, 66, 71
  see also Sun protection methods; Surgical remedies
Skin layers, 15
Skin types, 15–19, 21–22
Smoking
  effect on skin of, 65, 71
Soap
  effect on skin of, 26, 67
SPF see Sunscreens
Sport, 25, 32–33, 80
  see also Lifestyle
Squamous cell carcinoma, 56, 58–59
Sun damaged skin see Skin damage
Sun lamps see Tan
Sun Protection Factor (SPF) see Sunscreens
Sun protection methods, 23–34
Sun spots, 55
Sunburn, 35–40
  avoidance of, 39–40
  effects of, 38
Sunfilters see Sunscreens
Sunglasses, 41–44

Index

Sunscreens, 26–29
  application of, 29–30
  sensitivity to, 30–31, 39
  see also Creams; Make-up
Suntan *see* Tan
Surgical remedies, 49, 68–71
  see also Peeling, chemical peel
Swimming, 25
  see also Lifestyle; Sport

Tan, 12, 14, 21, 79
  chemical preparations for, 31
Trees, 32–33, 80

Ultraviolet radiation, 10, 17, 20–21, 27, 34, 35, 71, 81–84
  effect on immune system of, 22, 38, 50, 61–62
Umbrellas, 26, 75

Vitamin A, synthetic *see* Retinoid derivatives

Warts, 57
Water
  importance to health of, 71, 73, 76
Wrinkles, 44, 49, 65, 67, 68, 70